# REHABILITATION IN MENTAL HEALTH

## Goals and Objectives
## for Independent Living

Barbara J. Hemphill, MS, OTR, FAOTA

Cindee Quake Peterson, MA, OTR

Pamela Carr Werner, BS, OTR

**SLACK** Incorporated, 6900 Grove Road, Thorofare, New Jersey 08086-94

£64.99

Printed in the United States of America.

Library of Congress Catalog Card Number: 89-43121

Published by:    SLACK Incorporated
                 6900 Grove Road
                 Thorofare, NJ 08086 USA
                 Telephone: 856-848-1000
                 Fax: 856-853-5991
                 www.slackbooks.com

Contact SLACK Incorporated for more information about other books in this field or about the availability of our books from distributors outside the United States.

Last digit is print number: 10   9   8   7   6   5

# Dedication

*To the consumers of mental health services
who have the right to live as independently as possible.*

# Contents

# About the Authors

**Barbara J. Hemphill**

Barbara J. Hemphill is an associate professor in the Department of Occupational Therapy at Western Michigan University. Ms. Hemphill's publications include: **The Evaluative Process in Psychiatric Occupational Therapy, The B. H. Battery, Mental Health Assessment in Occupational Therapy, and Card File on Occupational Therapy Assesment in Mental Health.** Barbara has publications, research, and presentations in the areas of education, assessment, and mental health. She is a fellow of the American Occupational Therapy Association.

**Cindee Quake Peterson**

Cindee Quake Peterson is an assistant professor in the Occupational Therapy Department at Western Michigan University. She has worked in state and community mental health programs, and a residential treatment facility for emotionally disturbed children. She has also conducted Independent Living Skill Evaluations for community mental health boards, in accordance with Medicaid requirements. Cindee is currently an independent consultant for private human service businesses, and has publications in the areas of performance appraisal and pre-vocational assessment. Her recent research is in the use of robotics with the handicapped.

**Pamela Carr Werner**

Pamela Carr Werner is an occupational therapist in mental health and is the supervisor of a therapeutic work program at a psychiatric hospital in Kalamazoo, Michigan. She has been involved in numerous organizations including serving as board officer of the Michigan Chapter of the International Association of Psychosocial Rehabilitation Services. In addition, Pam has served as a trainer in the area of human resource development. She is an independent consultant to private human service businesses and has been a part-time faculty member in Western Michigan University's Occupational Therapy Department.

# Foreword

This book presents a logical model for clinical thinking and how to integrate professional health-care standards in order to establish realistic treatment programs for the psychiatrically impaired and effectively document treatment outcomes.

The writers identify the necessity for functional assessments and how these assessments affect the development of specific goals and objectives related to independent living skills for mental health patients. They identify three areas that need to be thoroughly evaluated and analyzed, namely: the performance components, barriers and maladaptive behaviors that are patient-related, and the behavioral tasks outlined under each independent living skill objective. The performance components are neuromotor (sensory, motor, neuromuscular, and motor functioning), cognitive, psychological and social.

Barriers include living arrangements and environments, length and type of hospitalization, family attitudes, and family understanding of the dynamics of the need for patient involvement. Maladaptive behaviors are those which interfere with learning and attaining independence. They are generally situation specific and may be related to diagnosis or medication effects. Behavioral tasks encompass the various jobs, chores, self-care activities, and acts which enable the individual to perform the independent living skills.

Appropriate evaluation of the performance components, barriers, and maladaptive behaviors identifies problem areas of dysfunction which will probably negate acquisition and performance of independent living skills. Each behavioral task must be analyzed (activity analysis) in relation to the performance components. This allows the therapist to match the outcome of the patient's assessment with a task that the patient has potential for performing, learning to perform it and integrating it as an ongoing daily life skill. Once the profile of the individual patient's performance levels and abilities is determined from these assessments, treatment goals and objectives can be set.

In today's health care delivery system, documentation of treatment outcome measures is required for receiving payment for services and in providing data relative to the efficacy of occupational therapy services. This text provides a simple but valid format for writing descriptive measurable goals and objectives and measurable outcomes in mental health. The Independent Living Skills chapters provide the component parts of an independent skill objective, namely: behavioral tasks, condition of performance, frequency of occurrence, criteria for moving to the next level, and time frame (all measurable). A very nice feature of these chapters is the very extensive list of behavioral skills indicated for each area. There are therapeutic suggestions for change at the end of each chapter.

A noteworthy aspect of this book is that the approach is applicable to the more severely involved and lower-level functioning patient. The process and behavioral tasks and skills depict the simple through the very complex. It is also an excellent format that is transferable to most patient populations. This book will serve as an excellent reference for both students and clinicians.

Nancy V. Snyder, MS, OTR/L, FAOTA
Assistant Clinical Professor
Occupational Therapy Division
School of Allied Health Professions
College of Medicine
The Ohio State University
President, American Occupational Therapy Foundation, 1985-1988

# Acknowledgements

The authors of the book would like to acknowledge Marianne McArthur, BS, OTR, for her suggestions, ideas, and input in the area of independent living skills; and Helen Diann Pratt, PhD, for her input, guidance, and technical assistance in how to write behavioral goals and objectives.

# Introduction

The purpose of this text is to provide a format for writing behavioral goals and objectives in the area of independent living skill acquisition. This text also assists the health care professional, para-professional, and student by providing a method for writing individualized treatment plans containing measurable goals, and suggests strategies to obtain these goals. Future prospective payment systems for reimbursement of health services mandate a systematic way of documenting and measuring treatment outcomes.

This textbook has a wide application to many impaired individuals who need to attain behavioral goals related to self-care, vocational, and leisure skills necessary for successful independent living. Often personality disorganization and maladaptive behaviors resulting from traumatic brain injury, developmental disability, and mental illness prevent acquisition of independent living skills.

The first three chapters in this book identify the need for a thorough assessment of performance prior to individualized goal setting. Chapter 1 looks at the "Performance Components" needed for independent living skill attainment. Performance components are identified as Neuro-motor, Cognitive, Psychological, and Social Skill areas necessary for community survival. Chapter 2 identifies how "Functional Assessments" are crucial in providing information needed for development of specific goals and objectives for independent living skill training programs. Data from functional assessments also provide objective information for billing purposes. Chapter 3, "Roadblocks to Skill Acquisition," provides an overview of barriers that may interfere with a client's ability to learn/relearn the performance components required for daily living.

Chapter 4, "How to Use This Book," identifies the format that the remaining chapters are based on, that is, how to write behavioral goals and objectives for independent living skills. A goal is defined and broken down into five components that are needed to formulate a behavioral objective. The component parts of a behavioral objective are the behavioral task, the condition of performance, the frequency of occurrence/duration, criteria for moving to the next level and the time frame for completion of the behavioral task. A grid format is used throughout the text to allow for a comprehensive listing of behavioral tasks, and provides cross-referenced examples of the five basic components needed to write a behavioral objective.

The remaining chapters are independent living skill chapters containing a brief description of a skill area such as "Dressing and Clothing Care, Chapter 6," a grid containing a comprehensive listing of behavioral tasks related to the skill area, the additional components needed to formulate a written behavioral objective and therapeutic suggestions that could be used to attain the behavioral task.

The skill chapters are in sequential order of when most independent living skills are learned developmentally, proceeding to a more advanced skill level needed for independent living. Skill chapters are presented in the following sequence: feeding, grooming, household management, leisure planning, social interaction, money management, community mobility, health-related behaviors, life-safety and work.

This book is intended to be a useful guide for the health care practitioner when documenting measurable goals and objectives for individualized treatment plans. The authors hope that this tool will assist in the documentation of appropriate treatment outcomes, and provide a method to attain increased accountability in training programs for independent living.

# Chapter 1

# Performance Components
## Stepping Stones to Skill Acquisition

The purpose of this chapter is to identify what skills, functions, or performances are needed for attainment of independent living skills for persons with mental illness. The need for an individualized functional assessment is emphasized in order to identify realistic goals and objectives for persons with psychiatric impairment.

Performance is defined as "a formal exhibition of skill" (Webster's New World Dictionary, 2nd ed.). Other key concepts describe performance as an "accomplishment," and refer to functioning as the "effectiveness" of performance.

The role of the health care professional is to determine what presenting problems prevent the individual with psychiatric impairment from attaining function, accomplishment, or performance in independent living. Prior to administering a functional assessment, one must look at independent living skills and determine what the client must be able to "do" if he is going to succeed in attaining the skill. The "do" part of performance can be described as the "component" or "step" needed to complete the skill.

Performance components are necessary skills to achieve the desired outcome or behavioral objective. The performance components give health care professionals an indication of where presenting problems exist so that intervention strategies can be implemented to achieve individualized goals. As part of the program planning process, the health care professional must assist the person with mental illness in learning the performance components that are missing or methods of adapting or substituting for the skill. In discussing specific goals and objectives necessary for independent living, one must thoroughly analyze which performance components are essential for each skill. The Neuro-motor, Cognitive, Psychological, and Social Skill areas are the performance components or "stepping stones" required for independent living skill acquisition.

## Neuro-motor Components

Neuro-motor components involve the sensory motor skills needed to respond to the environment. Vision, touch, hearing, taste, and the perceptual awareness of how to move muscles and negotiate through space are essential for functional performance.

### Table 1-1
### Neuro-motor Component

| Sensory Motor | Neuromuscular | Motor |
|---|---|---|
| sensory awareness | reflex | activity tolerance |
| tactile-touch | range of motion | coordination--gross and fine |
| proprioception | muscle tone | crossing midline |
| vestibular | strength | laterality |
| visual | endurance | bilateral integration |
| auditory | posture | praxis |
| taste | | dexterity |
| smell | | |
| stereognosis | | |
| kinesthesia | | |
| body scheme | | |
| R-L discrimination | | |
| form constancy | | |
| figure ground | | |
| depth perception | | |
| topographical orientation | | |

The individual who cannot discriminate hot from cold will be in jeopardy of burns. The one who has poor body image and does not have an understanding of where limbs are in space would be at risk at the jobsite. Neuro-motor deficits may be a side effect of medication which necessitates an evaluation by an occupational therapist to determine if the client truly presents a neurological problem. Areas to be evaluated include soft neurological signs, coordination, sensation, position in space, and visual perception. Table 1-1 identifies areas of neuro-motor performance required for independent living skills (Dunn & McGourty, 1989).

## Cognitive Components

Cognitive components allow for the decision making and problem solving needed to successfully engage in daily living. Cognition is a major predictor of independent living skill outcomes as identified by Claudia Allen, (1988), (1985), in her classification system of six cognitive levels of information processing by patients. These levels are used to observe and classify client functioning and can assist the health care professional in determining realistic goals and objectives regarding activities of daily living for persons with mental illness. Table 1-2 identifies areas of cognitive functioning required for independent living (Dunn & McGourty, 1989).

### Table 1-2
### Cognitive Integration and Cognitive Components

| | | |
|---|---|---|
| Level of arousal | Memory | Sequencing |
| Orientation | Synthesis of learning | Categorization |
| Recognition | | Concept formation |
| Attention | | Problems solving |
| Integration of learning | | Generalization of learning |

## Psychological Components

A problem often encountered by health care professionals in teaching functional skills to the person with mental illness is the lack of interest or motivation that the patient exhibits toward the activity. If the activity has no value or meaning for the patient, the activity is avoided or completed in a haphazard way. In addition, patients in mental health centers and psychiatric hospitals often demonstrate behaviors of pacing, hallucinating, talking to self, and delusions which can interfere with skill attainment. Determining an activity that will elicit the appropriate outcome is a difficult challenge with the psychiatric population. Knowledge of an individual's level of performance is essential in determining appropriate outcomes. Table 1-3 identifies the psychological skills for independent living (Dunn & McGourty, 1989).

### Table 1-3
### Psychological Components

| | |
|---|---|
| Roles | Initiation of activity |
| Values | Termination of activity |
| Interests | Self-concept |

## Social Components

Social conduct has had a major impact on the acquisition of independent living in the areas of self-maintenance, work, and leisure pursuits. Problems with re-entry of persons with mental illness into the community are society's expectations of the individual's role or adaptive behaviors and the value society places on the person's behaviors and skills (Reed & Sanderson, 1983, p. 51). A person who does not possess skills or performance components that are valued by society, or exhibits behaviors that do not meet social expectations may be shunned. Table 1-4 identifies social performance components needed for independent living (Dunn & McCourt, 1989).

### Table 1-4
### Social Components

| | |
|---|---|
| Social conduct | Coping skills |
| Conversation | Time management |
| Self-expression | Self-control |
| Self-management | |

## Conclusion

A functional assessment is an integral part of determining deficits in performance components, as well as a means to determine realistic expectations for attainment of independent living skills. Before the person with mental illness can be successfully integrated into the community, many independent living skill areas must be assessed. These may include, although are not limited to, accessing public transportation, community orientation, self-care, meal preparation, money management, household management, vocational exploration, and play or leisure exploration.

The following chapter will provide an overview of functional assessments that will assist in the development of specific goals and objectives for independent living.

# Chapter 2

# Functional Assessments

The purpose of this chapter is to provide an overview of how functional assessments affect the development of specific goals and objectives for independent living skill training programs; the functional assessment concept is defined and the importance of this assessment in relationship to treatment outcomes and accountability is discussed. A variety of functional assessments are listed to assist the mental health care professional in assessing recipients of mental health services.

Functional assessments are designed to evaluate the functioning level of a particular individual. Webster's New World Dictionary (second edition) defines functional as "performing or being able to perform a function, intended to be useful" and assessment as "to estimate or determine the significance, importance or value of." Therefore, functional assessment can be defined as a useful assessment that estimates or determines the performance of a specific function/task. An important word in this definition is the term useful. Some psychiatric assessments provide data that is interesting to read but not descriptive of the individual's behavior, skills, knowledge or strengths/limitations. A functional assessment provides data in these areas that is useful and effective in developing interdisciplinary treatment plans and outcomes. It may also provide information to assist the health care professional in determining the performance component areas of neuro-motor, cognitive, psychological and social that may require improvement for an individual to function at the highest level of independence. Before placing a client into a training program, it is important to provide a functional assessment in order to ensure that treatment provided is based on the performing level of the client.

A variety of health care professionals have recognized the importance of functional assessments in determining treatment that is outcome oriented. Denton (1988) reports that tracking the patient's functional ability helps to: a) assist in determining the diagnosis, b) monitor the effective medication and other treatments, c) determine problems in daily living, and d) identify supportive services and environment adaptations needed at discharge. Fine (1980) reports that the use of a functional assessment and evaluation of rehabilitation potential will provide information that is relevant to the discharge planning process. Allen (1988) states that the use of cognitive levels in functional assessment will help to determine: a) actions a client can perform, b) assistance needed to compensate for disabilities, c) severity of mental health disorder, d) changes in functional impairment over time or in response to treatment, e) need for hospitalization or community placement, f) readiness for discharge, and g) how the patient will function in the community. Furthermore, information from a functional assessment can be used to determine Axis V of the DSM III-R (Denton, 1988; Morrison, Fisher, Wilson, & Underwood, 1985). Axis V provides the clinician with the opportunity to indicate psychological, social and occupational functioning on a global assessment of functioning scale (DSM III-R, 1987). The scale requires two scores: 1) one regarding the current level of functioning and 2) a second score indicating the highest level of functioning in the past year. With the increase in accountability of treatment services, Axis V will continue to be utilized in determining functional levels and treatment services necessary to maintain or increase the level of adaptation in the hospital and/or community. Functional assessments provide objective data that can be utilized in an inpatient psychiatric setting to prepare clients for discharge and in the community to prevent future hospitalizations by determining the necessary supportive services needed to maintain or increase current level of functioning.

In addition to treatment and discharge planning, functional assessments are important and beneficial for administrative considerations. Many prospective payment systems (JCAHO, HCFA, Medicaid, and Medicare) continue to demand objective measures of outcome in psychiatric treatment in order to receive payment for treatment services rendered. Data from functional assessments provide objective information necessary for billing purposes. As prospective payment systems continue to demand accountability of treatment services, requirements for documentation of billable services will continue to increase. As treatment providers continue to contain costs for health care services in the United States, funds will be given to the health care providers who utilize treatment outcome measures and demonstrate clearly the impact and cost-effectiveness of their services (Carroll & Williams, 1982). As prospective payment systems continue to demand accountability for treatment services, the use of a functional assessment will assist in providing relevant data necessary to meet these demands.

A variety of functional assessments are available for health care professionals. Each assessment varies according to the behaviors and skill areas assessed. An alphabetical list of assessments provided in Table 2-1 may be helpful in developing an assessment program for in and outpatient treatment settings.

## Conclusion

In conclusion, this chapter provided an overview of functional assessments, including definitions, importance in developing treatment outcomes and validating cost-effective services. A list of functional assessments was provided to assist the health care professional in attaining a variety of assessments for the mental health population.

---

### Table 2-1
### Functional Assessments for Use by Health Professionals

| Functional Assessment | Purpose | Source |
|---|---|---|
| Allen Cognitive Levels (ACL) | Standard assessment intended to indicate the levels of independent living skills for the cognitively disabled. | Allen, C. K. (1985). *Occupational Therapy for Psychiatric Diseases: Measurement and Management of Cognitive Disabilities.* Boston: Little, Brown. |
| Comprehensive Evaluation of Basic Living Skills (CEBLS) | Battery of performance tests using checklist ratings. Evaluates wide range of daily living activities of varying complexity. Intended to indicate the functional status of chronic psychiatric patients. | Casanova, J. S. & Ferber, J. (1976). Comprehensive evaluation of basic living skills. *American Journal of Occupational Therapy*, 30, 101-105. |

## Table 2-1 (continued)

| Functional Assessments | Purpose | Source |
|---|---|---|
| Independent Living Behavior Checklist | Observation-based behavior checklist to determine skills needed for independent function. Based on institutionalized clients seeking an independent living situation. | West Virginia Rehabilitation Research and Training Center. |
| Independent Living Skills | Checklist involving interview and observation of performance. Comprehensive evaluation of skills needed for independent community living. Designed for chronically mentally disabled. | Johnson, Vinnicombe, & Merrill. (1980). The independent living skills evaluation. *Occupational Therapy in Mental Health*, (2). |
| Jacobs Pre-Vocational Assessment (JPVA) | Observation-based performance tasks designed to assess specific work-related skills in learning disabled adolescents. Applicable to chronic psychiatric patients. | Jacobs, K. (1985). *Occupational Therapy: Work-related Programs and Assessments*. Boston: Little, Brown. |
| Klein-Bell Activities of Daily Living Scale | Designed to provide a universally applicable measure of independence in activities of daily living. Although intended for use with most any population group, appears to be more physical disability oriented. | Health Sciences Learning Resource Center. |
| Kohlman Evaluation of Living Skills | Interview and task performance tool designed to provide a quick and simple evaluation of basic living skills. Intended for short-term psychiatric inpatients, although author suggests wider applications. | McGourty, L. (1988). *Kohlman Evaluation of Living Skills.* |
| Milwaukee Evaluation of Daily Living Skills (MEDLS) | Observation-based rating scale designed to provide a quantifiable measure of daily living skills for lower functioning, long-term psychiatric clients. | Leonardelli, C. A. (1988). *The Milwaukee Evaluation of Daily Living Skills: Evaluation in Long-term Psychiatric Care.* Thorofare, NJ: Slack, Inc. |

**Table 2-1 (continued)**

| Functional Assessments | Purpose | Source |
|---|---|---|
| Parachek Geriatric Rating Scale | Observation-based behavior rating scale intended to assist health care providers to group elderly patients by ability and potential. Areas addressed are physical, self-care, and social interaction skills. | Center for Neurodevelopmental Studies. |
| Scoreable Self-Care Evaluation | Standardized test based on observation, interview, and performance. Designed to provide a comprehensive measure of functional performance in basic living skills. Applicable for individuals with psychiatric disorders in acute and community settings. | Thorofare, NJ: Slack, Inc. |

From: Asher, I. E. (1989). *An Annotated Index of Occupational Therapy Evaluation Tools*. The American Occupational Therapy Association.

# Chapter 3

# Roadblocks to Skill Acquisition

The purpose of this chapter is to provide an overview of barriers that may interfere with the client's ability to learn/relearn the performance components required for independent living. Living arrangements that may encourage dependency are discussed. A list of maladaptive behaviors is provided in order to increase the health care professional's awareness of roadblocks that could interfere with the acquisition of independent living skills. The effect of these behaviors is related to performance components discussed in Chapter 1. This chapter concludes with a discussion of the importance of active involvement between the clinician and consumer in developing an individualized treatment program to increase the level of independent functioning.

Living arrangements can be a roadblock in the client's ability to acquire survival skills. Individuals with mental illness may require hospitalization for psychiatric treatment. When hospitalized, many of the skills necessary for independent functioning are performed by staff and care providers. Depending on the length of hospitalization, independent living skills may become forgotten as the opportunity to practice these important activities may not be available. If the living environment is not set up to encourage independence, often the expectations for the client are decreased or lowered. When observing clients in the process of performing independent living skills, it may appear that they are unable to complete the tasks. This could be related to the lack of opportunity and/or training provided to practice and learn activities of daily living. The opportunity to practice independent living skills can be a difficult problem in some community settings. Clients who live in Adult Foster Care (AFC) may be unable to learn the techniques of budgeting and cooking since home providers may complete these tasks themselves. In addition to hospitals and AFC providers, families

may not provide the opportunity to practice independent living skills. Without being aware of the consequences, family members may complete certain activities of daily living for the client since they verbalize inability or appear unable to complete the tasks themselves. Money may be budgeted for them, meals prepared, and prescriptions filled without their involvement in the active process. The living environment needs to be arranged to encourage self-sufficiency and increase behaviors necessary for community survival. The client may contribute to the dependency process by not becoming actively involved in completing daily living skills. It is easier to have others perform daily living activities than to complete them independently. When offered a choice, most people will select the behavior that requires the least amount of effort (Waley, Malott, & Garcia, in press). To encourage active involvement, the client must be included in decision making such as choosing the independent living skill training program and selecting the activity. The client's behavior must be reinforced immediately following the correct response to encourage active and continued involvement.

A variety of behaviors that appear as maladaptive could interfere with the client's ability to learn and attain independent living skills necessary for community survival. The health care professional should be aware of these competing behaviors when providing skill training. Table 3-1 presents an alphabetical list of some possible examples of behaviors that could interfere with skill acquisition.

Behaviors considered as maladaptive may be situation specific. For example, if an individual believes he/she is a millionaire and verbalizes this during an employment interview or refuses to complete any prevocational activities, then this behavior may be

## Table 3-1
## Conditions/Behaviors that Could
## Interfere with Skill Acquisition

| | | | |
|---|---|---|---|
| Acting out | Blocking | Flight of ideas | Phobias |
| Affect | Compliance | Grandiosity | Poor insight |
| Aggression | Compulsiveness | Hallucinations | Psychotic behavior |
| Agitation | Confusion | Impulsiveness | Self-esteem |
| Ambivalence | Delusions | Manipulation | Suicidal ideations |
| Anxiety | Dementia | Motivation | Withdrawn |
| Attention Span | Disorientation | Nonassertive | |
| Avoidance | Distractibility | Obsession | |

maladaptive. However, if this behavior arises when focusing on dressing and clothing care activities, it may not interfere with progress toward desired goals and objectives. When maladaptive behaviors interfere with goal attainment, then the treatment approach may require adaptations or special strategies.

In addition to maladaptive behaviors, other difficulties, such as physical impairments and the possible side effects of psychotropic medications, such as dizziness, drowsiness, tremors, and blurred vision should also be considered when developing an individualized treatment program. Table 3-2 provides a list of the side effects of psychotropic medications prescribed for persons with mental illnesses. It is important for both the client and health care provider to be aware of medication prescribed and possible side effects that may interfere with skill training.

Behaviors that appear as maladaptive may interfere with the ability to learn independent living skills, affecting the performance components needed to engage in activities of daily living, vocation, and leisure pursuits. When this occurs, the therapist can provide an enabler or treatment intervention to continue skill training.

When determining performance components needed for activities of daily living, the ability to process information may be limited if an individual has a short- or long-term memory deficit. For example, to learn the skills of functional mobility an individual

must be able to remember bus routes to successfully transfer to the desired location. If a memory deficit is assessed, the clinician may provide an enabler, treatment strategy, or adaptation to increase the level of independent functioning. One example may be to provide a written list of bus transfers required to reach the desired location.

Another example of a behavior that may impede the acquisition of daily living skills is confusion and disorientation. This behavior may interfere with skill training regarding medication knowledge and compliance. When an individual does not take his prescribed medication, this is labeled as a noncompliance problem. The noncompliant behavior may be a direct result of confusion or disorientation about the effect and type of the medication prescribed. If the recommended dosage is not explained to the client and/or written down, an increase in confusion may result, leading to noncompliant behaviors. Individuals who appear to have memory and cognitive deficits require simple one-and two-step directions or commands. Skill training requires adaptations with objectives written in smaller increments to measure goal progress and attainment.

When determining performance components for work activities, a variety of behaviors may interfere with skill acquisition. For instance, an individual may have a poor self-esteem which could interfere with the vocational activity of job acquisition. If you do not feel good about yourself, it is hard to describe to potential employers why you are the best candidate for the job. In order to facilitate the goal of job acquisition, the clinician must attend to the behavior of a low self-esteem and encourage verbalizations regarding positive self statements.

Performance components needed for play or leisure activities require social interaction skills. Withdrawn behaviors may interfere with the individual's ability to interact with his environment, family, or significant others. Before placing a client in a leisure program, the therapist may want to provide a treatment approach that directly addresses the withdrawn behaviors. Providing an environment that reinforces outgoing behaviors may increase the

## Table 3-2
## Side Effects of Psychotrophic Medications

| Drug | Purpose | Possible Side Effects |
|---|---|---|
| Elavil<br>Asendin<br>Norpramin<br>Pamelor<br>Sinequan<br>Trofanil | Prescribed to relieve depression and conditions including depression that occur with anxiety. | Dizziness<br>Drowsiness<br>Headache<br>Nausea<br>Unpleasant taste<br>Weight gain |
| Lithium | Prescribed to reduce the occurrence and severity of manic stages in manic depressive illness. | Diarrhea*<br>Drowsiness<br>Loss of appetite<br>Muscle weakness<br>Nausea or vomiting<br>Slurred speech<br>Trembling |
| Cogentin<br>Artane<br>Akineton | Prescribed for treatment of Parkinson's disease and to control severe reactions to certain drugs such as Navene, Loxitane, Haldol. | Clumsiness<br>Drowsiness<br>Shortness of breath<br>Blurred vision<br>Flushed skin |
| Haldol<br>Loxitane<br>Moban<br>Navane<br>Serentil<br>Mellaril<br>Stelazine<br>Prolixin<br>Thorazine | Prescribed for treatment of nervous, emotional, and mental conditions. | Blurred vision<br>Difficulty in swallowing or speaking<br>Loss of balance<br>Muscle spasm, especially face and neck<br>Restlessness<br>Shuffling walk<br>Chewing movements |
| Etrafon<br>Triavil | Prescribed for treatment of emotional and mental conditions. | Blurred vision<br>Difficulty in speaking or swallowing<br>Irregular heartbeat<br>Loss of balance<br>Muscle spasms, especially face and neck<br>Restlessness<br>Chewing movements |

*May be indicative of early warning signs of overdose
From United States Pharmacopeial Drug Information (1988). *Advice for Patient. 2.United States Pharmacopeial.*

client's ability to become more actively involved in leisure skill programming.

Before beginning an independent living skills training program, it is imperative that the client is involved in the active planning stages. The therapist and client must work together as a team to develop a plan that increases the level of independent functioning and acquisition of community-based survival skills.

For clients to become independent and self-sufficient, they require the opportunities, training, and positive reinforcement for their actions, efforts, and behaviors. The client should be able to visualize progress towards independent living skill accomplish-ments in order to increase participation and active involvement. Reinforcement for involvement and successful accomplishment is necessary to increase the client's motivational behaviors towards skill acquisition.

## Conclusion

This chapter provided an overview of roadblocks that may interfere with attaining survival skills that are necessary to increase independent functioning. It is important to assess maladaptive behaviors before placing an individual into an independent living skill curriculum in order to encourage successful accomplishments.

# Chapter 4

# How to Write Behavioral Goals and Objectives

The purpose of this chapter is to provide a suggested format on how to write behavioral goals and objectives in the area of independent living. This chapter will define and give examples of essential terms.

## Definition of a Goal

A goal is an expected outcome of a skill or task that is to be achieved over a period of time. Goals are typically broad in scope and provide guidance in developing objectives for skill attainment. They are often written in active statements such as increase, decrease, improve, report, participate, develop, and complete. The scope of goals needs to be determined by the skill level of the client.

## Definition of an Objective

Objectives are the smaller steps needed to accomplish the developed goal, and achieved over a shorter period of time. They often are stated in descriptive and measurable terms, achieved in a specific time frame and related to the attainment of a goal. Objectives need to encompass small samples of behavior to match the client's skill level and developed goal. Objectives have several components including:

A)      Behavioral task
B)      Condition of performance
C)      Frequency or Duration
D)      Criteria for moving to next level of performance
E)      Time frame

## Component Parts of an Objective

*Behavioral task:* Specifies the behavior or task that is to be learned. It needs to be written in positive and observable terms.

*Condition of performance:* Outlines what, where, and how an individual will demonstrate attainment of the objective.

*Frequency or duration:* Specifies how often or how long the behavior has to occur.

*Criteria for moving to next level:* Determines what steps must be completed before the next behavior or objective can be performed.

*Time frame:* Determines when behavior should be performed; state actual month, day, and year behavioral task should be completed.

## Example of a Goal and Objective

*Goal:* To improve work skills.

*Objective:*

a. **Behavioral task:** client will verbalize vocational strengths and weaknesses.
b. **Condition of performance:** with one verbal prompt.
c. **Frequency or duration:** 1 time per week.
d. **Criteria for moving to next level:** for six out of eight sessions (should include number or percent of consecutive successful trials).
e. **Time frame:** in 8 weeks (include month, day, and year).

Formulating goals and objectives in areas of independent living assists in developing an individualized treatment plan. Goals and objectives need to be written so that they can be realistically achieved by the client. They need to be stated in descriptive measurable terms so that client, family, and health care professional can understand the outcome and achievement dates. Table 4-1 provides a sample check list to determine if an objective contains the necessary component parts.

Measurable goals and objectives are important for assessing

client progress in activities of daily living and providing an accountable means for documenting the current status of functional performance. Careful measurement of an individual's functional level in independent living skills can provide the treatment team, prospective payment systems, accrediting organizations, and other related individuals or groups a way to determine if active treatment has been carried out.

The following chapters will incorporate component parts of an objective in a grid format. Once the goal is selected and behavioral task determined, components such as behaviorial task, condition of performance, frequency of occurrence or duration, criteria for moving to the next level, and time frame can be selected according to which components best fit the desired objective and the individual involved in the skill training program.

## Conclusion

This chapter provided an overview on how to write behavioral goals and objectives. The definitions of a goal and an objective were stated including the component parts that encompass objectives. A checklist was provided to assist the health care professional in determining whether a developed objective contains the necessary component parts. Finally, the importance of measurable goals and objectives was related to client progress, functional performance, and determination if active treatment has occurred.

**Table 4-1**
**Checklist for Component Parts of an Objective**

|  | Yes | No |
|---|---|---|
| 1. Is there a behavioral task? | ____ | ____ |
| a. Does it need to be learned? | ____ | ____ |
| b. Does it need to be strengthened? | ____ | ____ |
| c. Is it descriptive? | ____ | ____ |
| d. Is it observable? | ____ | ____ |
| e. Is it measurable? | ____ | ____ |
| 2. Is there a condition of performance? | ____ | ____ |
| a. Are environmental factors needed? | ____ | ____ |
| b. Are verbal prompts necessary? | ____ | ____ |
| c. Is physical guidance needed? | ____ | ____ |
| d. Are tactile cues necessary? | ____ | ____ |
| e. Will the behavior need to generalize to another setting? | ____ | ____ |
| 3. Is frequency or duration stated? | ____ | ____ |
| a. Is frequency needed? | ____ | ____ |
| b. Is duration needed? | ____ | ____ |
| 4. Is time frame stated? | ____ | ____ |
| a. Is the time or date of completion stated? | ____ | ____ |
| 5. Is the criteria for moving to the next level stated? | ____ | ____ |

# Chapter 5

# Food Consumption Activities

The purpose of this chapter is to list behavioral goals and objectives from the most "primitive" developmental levels regarding food consumption to more sophisticated objectives required for independent living. The ability to obtain and ingest food is the most primitive survival skill needed by all life forms. An individual must not only obtain and ingest food, but select the type and quality of food for healthy living. There are social and cultural mores attached to eating behaviors that can influence acceptance into the community at large. The following activities represent the multitude of behaviors that encompass the skill of food consumption.

**Eating** - Does the individual know the difference between edible and inedible objects? Does he differentiate between when to use utensils and when to use fingers, depending on the type of food and cultural influences?

**Table Manners** - Does the individual demonstrate socially acceptable behaviors of chewing with his mouth closed, using correct utensils and napkin, and placing the proper amount of food in his mouth so that it can be masticated without spilling?

Does the individual demonstrate an awareness of socially acceptable eating behaviors in public facilities, such as restaurants? Does the individual demonstrate an awareness of socially acceptable eating behaviors in the home environment?

**Food Preparation** - Is the individual aware of the five food groups and the necessity of including the five food groups in daily meals? Can the individual prepare a hot or cold meal? Does the individual demonstrate judgement through awareness of safety hazards when cooking, such as precautions when boiling water and using electrical appliances? Can he set a table using correct placement of utensils?

**Food Cleanup** - Can the individual clear the table and wash and dry dishes? Does he wipe up spills on countertops and appliances, clean a refrigerator, and dispose of spoiled food?

*Table 5-1*

| Food Consumption Activities | Objective | | | |
|---|---|---|---|---|
| **Behavioral Task** | **Condition of Performance** | **Frequency or Duration** | **Criteria for Moving to the Next Level of Performance** | **Time Frame** |
| **Eating.** The client will: | | | | |
| Discriminate between edible and inedible. | -with maximum physical guidance | 1 time per minute | 1 out of 3 times | by: (1 hour) |
| Open mouth in response to food stimulus. | -with moderate physical guidance | 3 times per minute | 3 out of 6 times | by: (6 hours) |
| Swallow food without spilling. | -with minimal physical guidance | 5 times per minute | __ out of __ times | by: (__ hours) |
| Swallow liquids without spilling. | - with ___% physical guidance | 1 time per hour | 4 consecutive trials out of 8 | by: (1 day) |
| Drink from straw. | - with tactile cues | 3 times per hour | 12 consecutive trials out of 15 | by: (3 days) |
| Drink from cup without spilling. | -with a demonstration | 5 times per hour | __ consecutive trials out of __ | by: (__ days) |
| Bring cup to mouth without spilling. | -with less than 5 verbal prompts | 6 consecutive times per hour | 20% of the time | by: (1 week) |
| Finger feed when appropriate. | -with less than 3 verbal prompts | 2 times per day | 50% of the time | by: (3 weeks) |
| Eat solid food with spoon without spilling. | -with 1 verbal prompt | 3 times per day | ___% of the time | by: (1 month) |
| Eat solid food with fork without spilling. | -with maximum assistance | 6 times per day | | by: (6 weeks) |
| Select appropriate utensil for food (knife, fork, spoon). | -with moderate assistance | 1 time per week | | by: (8 weeks) |
| | -with minimum assistance | 3 times per week | | by: (3 months) |
| Take adequate amount of food off utensil for appropriate chewing and to prevent choking. | -with ___% assistance | 8 times per week | | by: (__ months) |
| Cut with table knife in a safe manner. | -in the therapy setting | 1 time per month | | |
| **Table Manners.** The client will: | -in the home setting | 3 times per month | | |
| Wash hands using soap before meal. | -in a restaurant setting | 6 times per month | | © SLACK Inc. |
| | -independently | | | |

*Table 5-1 (Continued)*

| Food Consumption Activities | Objective | | | |
|---|---|---|---|---|
| **Behavioral Task** | **Condition of Performance** | **Frequency or Duration** | **Criteria for Moving to the Next Level of Performance** | **Time Frame** |
| Dry hands using towel. | -with maximum physical guidance | 1 time per minute | 1 out of 3 times | by: (1 hour) |
| Chew with mouth closed. | -with moderate physical guidance | 3 times per minute | 3 out of 6 times | by: (6 hours) |
| Recognize when to use a napkin. | -with minimal physical guidance | 5 times per minute | __ out of __ times | by: (__ hours) |
| Place napkin in lap before eating. | -with ___% physical guidance | 1 time per hour | 4 consecutive trials out of 8 | by: (1 day) |
| Wipe mouth with napkin when necessary. | -with tactile cues | 3 times per hour | 12 consecutive trials out of 15 | by: (3 days) |
| Pass food to others when requested. | -with a demonstration | 5 times per hour | __ consecutive trials out of __ | by: (__ days) |
| Request food from others. | -with less than 5 verbal prompts | 6 consecutive times per hour | 20% of the time | by: (1 week) |
| Take appropriate amount of portions from serving dishes. | -with less than 3 verbal prompts | 2 times per day | 50% of the time | by: (3 weeks) |
| Sit up straight at the table. | -with 1 verbal prompt | 3 times per day | ___% of the time | by: (1 month) |
| Keep elbows off the table during a meal. | -with maximum assistance | 6 times per day | | by: (6 weeks) |
| Talk without food in the mouth during a meal. | -with moderate assistance | 1 time per week | | by: (8 weeks) |
| Chew and swallow food before answering a question. | -with minimum assistance | 3 times per week | | by: (3 months) |
| | -with ___% assistance | 8 times per week | | by: (__ months) |
| Eat at a normal pace. | -in the therapy setting | 1 time per month | | |
| Practice appropriate dinner conversation. | -in the home setting | 3 times per month | | |
| Excuse self from table. | -independently | 6 times per month | | |
| | -safely | | | |

*Table 5-1 (Continued)*

| Food Consumption Activities | Objective | | | |
|---|---|---|---|---|
| **Behavioral Task** | **Condition of Performance** | **Frequency or Duration** | **Criteria for Moving to the Next Level of Performance** | **Time Frame** |
| **Food Preparation** | | | | |
| **Nutrition.** The client will: | -with maximum physical guidance | 1 time per minute | 1 out of 3 times | by: (1 hour) |
| Identify the five basic food groups (dairy, grains, fruit, vegetables and meat). | -with moderate physical guidance | 3 times per minute | 3 out of 6 times | by: (6 hours) |
| | -with minimal physical guidance | 5 times per minute | __ out of __ times | by: (__ hours) |
| Plan a balanced cold meal for self containing the five basic food groups. | -with ___% physical guidance | 1 time per hour | 4 consecutive trials out of 8 | by: (1 day) |
| Prepare a hot meal for self containing all five basic food groups. | -with tactile cues | 3 times per hour | 12 consecutive trials out of 15 | by: (3 days) |
| | -with a demonstration | 5 times per hour | __ consecutive trials out of __ | by: (__ days) |
| Plan a daily menu including the five basic food groups. | -with less than 5 verbal prompts | 6 consecutive times per hour | 20% of the time | by: (1 week) |
| Plan a weekly menu including the five basic food groups. | -with less than 3 verbal prompts | 2 times per day | 50% of the time | by: (3 weeks) |
| | -with 1 verbal prompt | 3 times per day | ___% of the time | by: (1 month) |
| Identify non-nutritious foods. | -with maximum assistance | 6 times per day | | by: (6 weeks) |
| Limit non-nutritious foods in daily menu. | -with moderate assistance | 1 time per week | | by: (8 weeks) |
| Read ingredient labels to determine if food products are nutritious. | -with minimum assistance | 3 times per week | | by: (3 months) |
| | -with ___% assistance | 8 times per week | | by: (__ months) |
| **Preparation.** The client will: | -in the therapy setting | 1 time per month | | |
| Set table with appropriate placement of utensils. | -in the home setting | 3 times per month | | |
| Make a sandwich. | -independently | 6 times per month | | |
| Prepare a bowl of cold cereal. | -safely | | | |

© SLACK Inc.

18

*Table 5-1 (Continued)*

| Food Consumption Activities | Objective | | | |
|---|---|---|---|---|
| **Behavioral Task** | **Condition of Performance** | **Frequency or Duration** | **Criteria for Moving to the Next Level of Performance** | **Time Frame** |
| Open packages and containers without spilling. | -with maximum physical guidance | 1 time per minute | 1 out of 3 times | by: (1 hour) |
| Open cans with a can opener (electric or handheld) without spilling. | -with moderate physical guidance | 3 times per minute | 3 out of 6 times | by: (6 hours) |
| Turn on gas or electric stove/oven. | -with minimal physical guidance | 5 times per minute | __ out of __ times | by: (__ hours) |
| Consistently turn off gas or electric stove/oven following use. | -with ___% physical guidance | 1 time per hour | 4 consecutive trials out of 8 | by: (1 day) |
| Light gas with match. | -with tactile cues | 3 times per hour | 12 consecutive trials out of 15 | by: (3 days) |
| Peel vegetables in a safe manner. | -with a demonstration | 5 times per hour | __ consecutive trials out of __ | by: (__ days) |
| Wash produce before eating. | -with less than 5 verbal prompts | 6 consecutive times per hour | 20% of the time | by: (1 week) |
| Cut vegetables in a safe manner using a kitchen knife. | -with less than 3 verbal prompts | 2 times per day | 50% of the time | by: (3 weeks) |
| Use a bottle opener. | -with 1 verbal prompt | 3 times per day | ___% of the time | by: (1 month) |
| Handle sharp kitchen utensils safely. | -with maximum assistance | 6 times per day | | by: (6 weeks) |
| Break an egg. | -with moderate assistance | 1 time per week | | by: (8 weeks) |
| Pour hot water safely into containers (cup). | -with minimum assistance | 3 times per week | | by: (3 months) |
| Make a cup of instant coffee. | -with ___% assistance | 8 times per week | | by: (__ months) |
| Make a cup of coffee in a coffee maker. | -in the therapy setting | 1 time per month | | |
| Follow boxed instructions for correct | -in the home setting | 3 times per month | | |
| | -independently | 6 times per month | | |
| | -safely | | | |

© SLACK Inc.

*Table 5-1 (Continued)*

| *Food Consumption Activities* | **Objective** | | | |
|---|---|---|---|---|
| **Behavioral Task** | **Condition of Performance** | **Frequency or Duration** | **Criteria for Moving to the Next Level of Performance** | **Time Frame** |
| Follow instructions on cans for correct sequence of food preparation. | -with maximum physical guidance | 1 time per minute | 1 out of 3 times | by: (1 hour) |
| | -with moderate physical guidance | 3 times per minute | 3 out of 6 times | by: (6 hours) |
| Cook simple hot foods such as eggs, soup, or macaroni and cheese. | -with minimal physical guidance | 5 times per minute | __ out of __ times | by: (__ hours) |
| Prepare frozen foods following instructions for microwave. | -with ___% physical guidance | 1 time per hour | 4 consecutive trials out of 8 | by: (1 day) |
| | -with tactile cues | 3 times per hour | 12 consecutive trials out of 15 | by: (3 days) |
| Prepare frozen foods following instructions for oven. | -with a demonstration | 5 times per hour | __ consecutive trials out of __ | by: (__ days) |
| Prepare TV dinners following instructions for microwave. | -with less than 5 verbal prompts | 6 consecutive times per hour | 20% of the time | by: (1 week) |
| | -with less than 3 verbal prompts | 2 times per day | 50% of the time | by: (3 weeks) |
| Prepare TV dinners following instructions for oven. | -with 1 verbal prompt | 3 times per day | ___% of the time | by: (1 month) |
| Fry items safely on the stove. | -with maximum assistance | 6 times per day | | by: (6 weeks) |
| Safely drain grease from pan into a container. | -with moderate assistance | 1 time per week | | by: (8 weeks) |
| Boil items safely on the stove. | -with minimum assistance | 3 times per week | | by: (3 months) |
| Use hand mitts or pot holders when cooking. | -with ___% assistance | 8 times per week | | by: (__ months) |
| Wear safe clothing when cooking (no dangling scarves, etc.) | -in the therapy setting | 1 time per month | | |
| | -in the home setting | 3 times per month | | |
| Use a toaster. | -independently | 6 times per month | | |
| Use an electric frying pan. | -safely | | | |
| Use a microwave oven. | | | | |

*Table 5-1 (Continued)*

| *Food Consumption Activities* | **Objective** | | | |
|---|---|---|---|---|
| **Behavioral Task** | **Condition of Performance** | **Frequency or Duration** | **Criteria for Moving to the Next Level of Performance** | **Time Frame** |
| Use an electric mixer. | -with maximum physical guidance | 1 time per minute | 1 out of 3 times | by: (1 hour) |
| Follow and cook a pictorial recipe that has 3 ingredients. | -with moderate physical guidance | 3 times per minute | 3 out of 6 times | by: (6 hours) |
| Follow and cook a pictorial recipe that has 5 ingredients. | -with minimal physical guidance | 5 times per minute | __ out of __ times | by: (__ hours) |
|  | -with ___% physical guidance | 1 time per hour | 4 consecutive trials out of 8 | by: (1 day) |
| Follow and cook a recipe, that has 3 ingredients, using measuring cups or spoons. | -with tactile cues | 3 times per hour | 12 consecutive trials out of 15 | by: (3 days) |
|  | -with a demonstration | 5 times per hour | __ consecutive trials out of __ | by: (__ days) |
| Follow and cook a recipe, that has 5 ingredients, using measuring cups or spoons. | -with less than 5 verbal prompts | 6 consecutive times per hour | 20% of the time | by: (1 week) |
| Follow and cook a recipe in a standard cookbook. | -with less than 3 verbal prompts | 2 times per day | 50% of the time | by: (3 weeks) |
| Prepare a shopping list for at least 3 items from a grocery store. | -with 1 verbal prompt | 3 times per day | ___% of the time | by: (1 month) |
|  | -with maximum assistance | 6 times per day |  | by: (6 weeks) |
| Prepare a shopping list for at least 10 items from a grocery store. | -with moderate assistance | 1 time per week |  | by: (8 weeks) |
|  | -with minimum assistance | 3 times per week |  | by: (3 months) |
| Plan, prepare, and serve a hot meal for more than 2 people. | -with ___% assistance | 8 times per week |  | by: (__ months) |
| Plan and prepare balanced meals for self on a regular basis. | -in the therapy setting | 1 time per month |  |  |
| **Food Cleanup.** The client will: | -in the home setting | 3 times per month |  |  |
| Clear table of dishes. | -independently | 6 times per month |  |  |
| Scrape plates of any garbage and dispose in appropriate trash container. | -safely |  |  |  |

*Table 5-1 (Continued)*

| Food Consumption Activities | Objective | | | |
|---|---|---|---|---|

| Behavioral Task | Condition of Performance | Frequency or Duration | Criteria for Moving to the Next Level of Performance | Time Frame |
|---|---|---|---|---|
| Store leftover food in correct containers following meal and refrigerate, if necessary. | -with maximum physical guidance | 1 time per minute | 1 out of 3 times | by: (1 hour) |
| | -with moderate physical guidance | 3 times per minute | 3 out of 6 times | by: (6 hours) |
| Fill kitchen sink with liquid detergent and water. | -with minimal physical guidance | 5 times per minute | __ out of __ times | by: (__ hours) |
| Use proper amount of liquid detergent. | -with ___% physical guidance | 1 time per hour | 4 consecutive trials out of 8 | by: (1 day) |
| Hand wash the dishes. | -with tactile cues | 3 times per hour | 12 consecutive trials out of 15 | by: (3 days) |
| Hand rinse the dishes. | -with a demonstration | 5 times per hour | __ consecutive trials out of __ | by: (__ days) |
| Place rinsed dishes in drain rack. | -with less than 5 verbal prompts | 6 consecutive times per hour | 20% of the time | by: (1 week) |
| Empty kitchen sink of wash and rinse water. | -with less than 3 verbal prompts | 2 times per day | 50% of the time | by: (3 weeks) |
| Dry the dishes. | -with 1 verbal prompt | 3 times per day | ___% of the time | by: (1 month) |
| Place dishes in correct cupboards. | -with maximum assistance | 6 times per day | | by: (6 weeks) |
| Clean off counters and table with a damp cloth or sponge following the meal. | -with moderate assistance | 1 time per week | | by: (8 weeks) |
| | -with minimum assistance | 3 times per week | | by: (3 months) |
| Scrub off or rinse dishes under faucet before placing in dishwasher. | -with ___% assistance | 8 times per week | | by: (__ months) |
| Load a dishwasher. | -in the therapy setting | 1 time per month | | |
| Place dishwasher detergent in the appropriate opening. | -in the home setting | 3 times per month | | |
| Operate the controls on a dishwasher. | -independently | 6 times per month | | |
| Scrub kitchen sink using correct cleanser. | -safely | | | |

© SLACK Inc.

22

*Table 5-1 (Continued)*

| Food Consumption Activities | Objective | | | |
| --- | --- | --- | --- | --- |

| Behavioral Task | Condition of Performance | Frequency or Duration | Criteria for Moving to the Next Level of Performance | Time Frame |
| --- | --- | --- | --- | --- |
| Wipe off front of stove, refrigerator,microwave, coffee pot, toaster, etc., following use. | -with maximum physical guidance | 1time per minute | 1 out of 3 times | by: (1hour) |
| | -with moderate physical guidance | 3 times per minute | 3 out of 6 times | by: (6 hours) |
| Clean kitchen floor of any spilled food following meal. | -with minimal physical guidance | 5 times per minute | __ out of __ times | by: (__ hours) |
| | -with ___% physical guidance | 1 time per hour | 4 consecutive trials out of 8 | by: (1 day) |
| Take garbage out to trash can. | -with tactile cues | 3 times per hour | 12 consecutive trials out of 15 | by: (3 days) |
| Clean out trash containers and line with paper sacks or plastic garbage bags. | -with a demonstration | 5 times per hour | __ consecutive trials out of __ | by: (__ days) |
| **Food Spoilage.** The client will: | -with less than 5 verbal prompts | 6 consecutive times per hour | 20% of the time | by: (1 week) |
| Demonstrate an understanding of the shelf-life of food products. | -with less than 3 verbal prompts | 2 times per day | 50% of the time | by: (3 weeks) |
| Identify the date that refrigerated food should be consumed by. | -with 1 verbal prompt | 3 times per day | ___% of the time | by: (1 month) |
| | -with maximum assistance | 6 times per day | | by: (6 weeks) |
| Consistently check refrigerated food for spoilage. | -with moderate assistance | 1 time per week | | by: (8 weeks) |
| | -with minimum assistance | 3 times per week | | by: (3 months) |
| Dispose of spoiled food in the refrigerator and cupboards regularly. | -with ___% assistance | 8 times per week | | by: (__ months) |
| | -in the therapy setting | 1 time per month | | |
| prior to refrigerating. | -in the home setting | 3 times per month | | |
| | -independently | 6 times per month | | |

## Therapeutic Suggestions

1. Use a mirror during feeding to show the client a correct body posture. Mirrors are also important media to show the client appropriate ways to chew and socially appropriate ingestion of amount of food by calling to his attention how he looks to others while eating. (Mirrors may not be helpful to individuals who cannot voluntarily control their oral-motor movement.)

2. Videotape the client using various utensils, and have the client critique his skill. Give verbal prompts as to the amount of food that can be safely handled on the utensil.

3. Talk about various types of food and have the client identify which ones can be eaten with fingers in public and which ones require the use of utensils.

4. Talk about a variety of foods, and have the client identify which utensil would be the best choice for eating the food. (Example: using a spoon versus a fork for jello.)

5. Design a pictorial aide on cleaning and defrosting the refrigerator.

6. Talk about what type of cleaners to use for sinks, counter tops, stoves, refrigerators, and dishes, and how to accomplish the task of cleaning appliances.

7. Talk about and practice reading labels on foods to determine by what date the food should be consumed.

8. Talk about what spoiled food looks like and what can happen if it is ingested (food poisoning).

9. Develop a daily meal planner or log of menus for breakfast, lunch, and dinner incorporating the correct amounts of the five basic food groups.

10. Make color-coded food cards of the basic food groups (five different colors) and plan meals using a card from each food group for each meal.

11. Practice reading ingredient labels on foods to determine if the food product includes vitamins and minerals needed on a daily basis.

12. Practice reading ingredient labels on food to determine the amount of non-nutritious substances such as sugar content and sodium. Practice selecting items that are low fat, low cholesterol, low sodium, and with no preservatives.

13. Have the client make a pictorial cookbook on their favorite dishes and add recipes with pictures cut from magazines.

14. Provide information on the minimum kitchen aides needed for apartment living and prioritize items that are the most important, such as a can opener.

15. Provide pictorial aides in measuring and what utensils to use for measurement.

16. Practice reading a measuring cup.

17. Practice reading measuring spoons.

18. Run a cooking group and make a full meal. Invite guests and practice dinner conversation.

19. Run a nutrition group and discuss the amount, type, and kind of food to eat each day.

20. Have all group members bring sack lunches to group. Have each member determine the fat and calorie content of his lunch and discuss which group member has the most nutritious meal.

21. Have group members demonstrate appropriate and non-appropriate table manners. Videotape a meal and have members critique their table manners and make suggestions on how they can improve them.

22. Run a meal planning group and have all members develop a shopping list, go to the store, and compare prices and discuss best values.

23. Know where community resources are located on consumer nutrition (American Heart Association) and get information on nutrition for client groups.

24. Have group members prepare a meal and sit down to eat it together. As group leader, concentrate on identifying the pacing of the group. Ask each member to taste all servings individually, ask for seconds appropriately, pass dishes to the left, etc.

# Chapter 6

# Dressing and Clothing Care

The purpose of this chapter is to identify dressing and clothing care activities essential for independent living. Clothing provides a means of expressing individuality and personality. The clothing that we wear gives clues to other people about our careers, socio-economic status, grooming habits, and concern for personal appearance. The trend toward de-institutionalization for the mentally ill has placed many individuals into the community who may stand out as being "abnormal" or "different," based entirely on how they are dressed. Unfortunately, individuals are typically judged by personal appearance first, and then by other factors which can be handicapping influences for the chronically mentally ill. It is essential that health care professionals assist the mentally ill into community reintegration by "normalizing" appearance through appropriate dressing and clothing care. The following activities represent the multitude of behaviors necessary for dressing and clothing care.

**Dressing** - Can the client dress himself without assistance? Does he dress for weather related conditions? Can he open and close fasteners or attend to these when dressing (pants without belt, zippers left open)? Does he wear the appropriate size of clothing (pants too short, pants too large around waist)? Does he wear appropriate colors and patterns together (stripes with polka dots)? Can he identify soiled clothing? Does he assume responsibility for washing clothing or directing attention to soiled clothing that requires cleaning (placing in hamper)? Can he repair minor tears or lost buttons? Can he shop for clothing and identify correct size and clothing care instructions (dry clean, hand wash, machine wash-- cold)?

*Table 6-1*

| Dressing and Clothing Care | **Objective** | | | |
|---|---|---|---|---|
| **Behavioral Task** | **Condition of Performance** | **Frequency or Duration** | **Criteria for Moving to the Next Level of Performance** | **Time Frame** |
| **Dressing.** The client will: | | | | |
| Identify back from front of clothing. | -with maximum physical guidance | 1 time per minute | 1 out of 3 times | by: (1 hour) |
| Identify inside from outside of clothing. | -with moderate physical guidance | 3 times per minute | 3 out of 6 times | by: (6 hours) |
| Identify top from bottom of clothing. | -with minimal physical guidance | 5 times per minute | ___ out of ___ times | by: (___ hours) |
| Identify sequence of dressing (socks before shoes, underwear before pants). | -with ___% physical guidance | 1 time per hour | 4 consecutive trials out of 8 | by: (1 day) |
| | -with tactile cues | 3 times per hour | 12 consecutive trials out of 15 | by: ( 3 days) |
| Identify arm holes and leg holes in clothing. | -with a demonstration | 5 times per hour | ___ consecutive trials out of ___ | by: (___ days) |
| Dress the correct body part (arms in shirts, pants on legs). | -with less than 5 verbal prompts | 6 consecutive times per hour | 20% of the time | by: (1 week) |
| Remove all clothing when undressing. | -with less than 3 verbal prompts | 2 times per day | 50% of the time | by: (3 weeks) |
| Put on all appropriate clothing. | -with 1 verbal prompt | 3 times per day | ___% of the time | by: (1 month) |
| Place shoes on the correct feet. | -with maximum assistance | 6 times per day | | by: (6 weeks) |
| Thread a belt through belt loops correctly. | -with moderate assistance | 1 time per week | | by: (8 weeks) |
| **Unfastening.** The client will: | -with minimum assistance | 3 times per week | | by: (3 months) |
| Unbutton clothing. | -with ___% assistance | 8 times per week | | by: (___ months) |
| Unzip clothing. | -in the therapy setting | 1 time per month | | |
| Untie clothing/shoes. | -in the home setting | 3 times per month | | |
| Unhook clothing. | -independently | 6 times per month | | |
| Unsnap clothing. | | | | |
| Unbuckle clothing/belt. | | | | |
| Unfasten velcro tabs. | | | | © SLACK Inc. |

*Table 6-1 (Continued)*

| Dressing and Clothing Care | **Objective** | | | |
|---|---|---|---|---|
| **Behavioral Task** | **Condition of Performance** | **Frequency or Duration** | **Criteria for Moving to the Next Level of Performance** | **Time Frame** |
| **Fastening.** The client will: | | | | |
| Line up fasteners correctly. | -with maximum physical guidance | 1 time per minute | 1 out of 3 times | by: (1 hour) |
| Button clothing for correct closure. | -with moderate physical guidance | 3 times per minute | 3 out of 6 times | by: (6 hours) |
| Tie clothing and shoes for correct closure. | -with minimal physical guidance | 5 times per minute | __ out of __ times | by: (__ hours) |
| Zip clothing for correct closure. | -with ___% physical guidance | 1 time per hour | 4 consecutive trials out of 8 | by: (1 day) |
| Hook clothing for correct closure. | -with tactile cues | 3 times per hour | 12 consecutive trials out of 15 | by: (3 days) |
| Snap clothing for correct closure. | -with a demonstration | 5 times per hour | __ consecutive trials out of __ | by: (__ days) |
| Buckle clothing and belts for correct closure. | -with less than 5 verbal prompts | 6 consecutive times per hour | 20% of the time | by: (1 week) |
| Fasten velcro tabs for correct closure. | -with less than 3 verbal prompts | 2 times per day | 50% of the time | by: (3 weeks) |
| **Clothes Selection and Maintenance.** The client will: | -with 1 verbal prompt | 3 times per day | ___% of the time | by: (1 month) |
| | -with maximum assistance | 6 times per day | | by: (6 weeks) |
| Select and wear correct clothing for weather conditions (sweater for cool weather, sandals for warm weather). | -with moderate assistance | 1 time per week | | by: (8 weeks) |
| | -with minimum assistance | 3 times per week | | by: (3 months) |
| Look into mirror to adjust clothing on person so there are no wrinkles and that correct fit is maintained. | -with ___% assistance | 8 times per week | | by: (__ months) |
| | -in the therapy setting | 1 time per month | | |
| Select and wear correct clothing for color and pattern. | -in the home setting | 3 times per month | | |
| | -in a community setting | 6 times per month | | |
| | -independently | | | |

*Table 6-1 (Continued)*

| Dressing and Clothing Care | | | Objective | | |
|---|---|---|---|---|---|

| Behavioral Task | Condition of Performance | Frequency or Duration | Criteria for Moving to the Next Level of Performance | Time Frame |
|---|---|---|---|---|
| Select and wear clean clothing. | -with maximum physical guidance | 1 time per minute | 1 out of 3 times | by: (1 hour) |
| Discriminate between neat, complete dressing versus sloppy, incomplete dressing. | -with moderate physical guidance | 3 times per minute | 3 out of 6 times | by: (6 hours) |
|  | -with minimal physical guidance | 5 times per minute | __ out of __ times | by: (__ hours) |
| Discriminate between soiled and unsoiled clothing. | -with ___% physical guidance | 1 time per hour | 4 consecutive trials out of 8 | by: (1 day) |
| Discriminate between outdated clothing and current clothing. | -with tactile cues | 3 times per hour | 12 consecutive trials out of 15 | by: (3 days) |
|  | -with a demonstration | 5 times per hour | __ consecutive trials out of __ | by: (__ days) |
| Identify correct size of clothing for purchase. | -with less than 5 verbal prompts | 6 consecutive times per hour | 20% of the time | by: (1 week) |
| Wear correct size of clothing. | -with less than 3 verbal prompts | 2 times per day | 50% of the time | by: (3 weeks) |
| Identify clothing tags for care (hand wash, dry clean, etc.). | -with 1 verbal prompt | 3 times per day | ___% of the time | by: (1 month) |
| Identify clothing tags for care (cotton, wool, linen). | -with maximum assistance | 6 times per day |  | by: (6 weeks) |
|  | -with moderate assistance | 1 time per week |  | by: (8 weeks) |
| Try on clothing for fit. | -with minimum assistance | 3 times per week |  | by: (3 months) |
| Identify if clothing fits correctly (pants too short, too big). | -with ___% assistance | 8 times per week |  | by: (__ months) |
| Identify if clothing is affordable. | -in the therapy setting | 1 time per month |  |  |
| Identify need to purchase clothing and verbalize this to primary care provider, payee, or significant other. | -in the home setting | 3 times per month |  |  |
|  | -independently | 6 times per month |  |  |
| Purchase clothing according to size, fit, affordability, and ease in cleaning. | -in a store setting |  |  |  |

*Table 6-1 (Continued)*

| Dressing and Clothing Care | Objective | | | |
|---|---|---|---|---|
| **Behavioral Task** | **Condition of Performance** | **Frequency or Duration** | **Criteria for Moving to the Next Level of Performance** | **Time Frame** |
| Select and buy appropriate size of clothing. | -with maximum physical guidance | 1 time per minute | 1 out of 3 times | by: (1 hour) |
| Identify stores to shop for less expensive clothing. | -with moderate physical guidance | 3 times per minute | 3 out of 6 times | by: (6 hours) |
| **Laundry.** The client will: | -with minimal physical guidance | 5 times per minute | __ out of __ times | by: (__ hours) |
| Identify frequency of changing undergarments and clothing for cleanliness. | -with ___% physical guidance | 1 time per hour | 4 consecutive trials out of 8 | by: (1 day) |
| | -with tactile cues | 3 times per hour | 12 consecutive trials out of 15 | by: (3 days) |
| Identify soiled clothes. | -with a demonstration | 5 times per hour | __ consecutive trials out of __ | by: (__ days) |
| Place soiled clothing in laundry hamper. | -with less than 5 verbal prompts | 6 consecutive times per hour | 20% of the time | by: (1 week) |
| Read clothing tags for wash and temperature cycle. | -with less than 3 verbal prompts | 2 times per day | 50% of the time | by: (3 weeks) |
| Sort light clothing from dark clothing. | -with 1 verbal prompt | 3 times per day | ___% of the time | by: (1 month) |
| Sort laundry needing dry cleaning. | -with maximum assistance | 6 times per day | | by: (6 weeks) |
| Check pockets of clothing before laundering. | -with moderate assistance | 1 time per week | | by: (8 weeks) |
| Follow instructions for loading the washing machine. | -with minimum assistance | 3 times per week | | by: (3 months) |
| | -with ___% assistance | 8 times per week | | by: (__ months) |
| Place soiled clothing in washing machine. | -in the therapy setting | 1 time per month | | |
| Use appropriate amount of laundry detergent/bleach/fabric softener in washing machine. | -in the home setting | 3 times per month | | |
| Select appropriate wash and rinse temperature on the washing machine. | -independently | 6 times per month | | |

© SLACK Inc.

31

*Table 6-1 (Continued)*

| Dressing and Clothing Care | Objective | | | |
|---|---|---|---|---|
| **Behavioral Task** | **Condition of Performance** | **Frequency or Duration** | **Criteria for Moving to the Next Level of Performance** | **Time Frame** |
| Select appropriate water level on washing machine. | -with maximum physical guidance | 1 time per minute | 1 out of 3 times | by: (1 hour) |
| Select appropriate wash cycle on washing machine. | -with moderate physical guidance | 3 times per minute | 3 out of 6 times | by: (6 hours) |
| | -with minimal physical guidance | 5 times per minute | __ out of __ times | by: (__ hours) |
| Operate the controls on a washing machine. | -with ___% physical guidance | 1 time per hour | 4 consecutive trials out of 8 | by: (1 day) |
| Place clothing in dryer. | -with tactile cues | 3 times per hour | 12 consecutive trials out of 15 | by: (3 days) |
| Select appropriate temperature and time on the dryer. | -with a demonstration | 5 times per hour | __ consecutive trials out of __ | by: (__ days) |
| Operate the controls on a dryer. | -with less than 5 verbal prompts | 6 consecutive times per hour | 20% of the time | by: (1 week) |
| Identify when clothes are dry. | -with less than 3 verbal prompts | 2 times per day | 50% of the time | by: (3 weeks) |
| Clean dryer lint trap as needed. | -with 1 verbal prompt | 3 times per day | ___% of the time | by: (1 month) |
| Fold clothing and place in drawers. | -with maximum assistance | 6 times per day | | by: (6 weeks) |
| Hang appropriate clothing in closet. | -with moderate assistance | 1 time per week | | by: (8 weeks) |
| Hand wash and rinse appropriate clothing items using soap. | -with minimum assistance | 3 times per week | | by: (3 months) |
| | -with ___% assistance | 8 times per week | | by: (__ months) |
| Operate a coin-operated washing machine and dryer. | -in the therapy setting | 1 time per month | | |
| | -in the home setting | 3 times per month | | |
| **Clothing Repair.** The client will: | -in a community setting | 6 times per month | | |
| Identify torn or damaged clothing. | -independently | | | |
| Identify need to replace a button on clothing. | | | | |

© SLACK Inc.

*Table 6-1 (Continued)*

| *Dressing and Clothing Care* | **Objective** | | | |
|---|---|---|---|---|
| **Behavioral Task** | **Condition of Performance** | **Frequency or Duration** | **Criteria for Moving to the Next Level of Performance** | **Time Frame** |
| Select correct size button to sew on clothing. | -with maximum physical guidance | 1 time per minute | 1 out of 3 times | by: (1 hour) |
| Select correct color of thread to sew on button. | -with moderate physical guidance | 3 times per minute | 3 out of 6 times | by: (6 hours) |
| Sew on a button. | -with minimal physical guidance | 5 times per minute | __ out of __ times | by: (__ hours) |
| Repair minor damage to clothing such as tears or fallen hems. | -with ___% physical guidance | 1 time per hour | 4 consecutive trials out of 8 | by: (1 day) |
| Identify to supportive other clothing in need of repair. | -with tactile cues | 3 times per hour | 12 consecutive trials out of 15 | by: (3 days) |
| | -with a demonstration | 5 times per hour | __ consecutive trials out of __ | by: (__ days) |
| Discard clothing damaged beyond repair. | -with less than 5 verbal prompts | 6 consecutive times per hour | 20% of the time | by: (1 week) |
| | -with less than 3 verbal prompts | 2 times per day | 50% of the time | by: (3 weeks) |
| **Ironing.** The client will: | -with 1 verbal prompt | 3 times per day | ___% of the time | by: (1 month) |
| Obtain equipment needed for ironing (board, iron, spray starch, spray bottle). | -with maximum assistance | 6 times per day | | by: (6 weeks) |
| Identify when purchasing clothes what fabrics will require ironing. | -with moderate assistance | 1 time per week | | by: (8 weeks) |
| Identify when clothing requires ironing. | -with minimum assistance | 3 times per week | | by: (3 months) |
| Set temperature of iron for clothing fabric. | -with ___% assistance | 8 times per week | | by: (__ months) |
| Iron clothing safely. | -in the therapy setting | 1 time per month | | |
| Iron clothing front and back. | -in the home setting | 3 times per month | | |
| Hang ironed article on hanger. | -independently | 6 times per month | | |
| Unplug iron and put it away following use. | | | | |
| Put ironing board away following use. | | | | |

© SLACK Inc.

## Therapeutic Suggestions

1. Cut out pictures from magazines of individuals who look well dressed versus individuals who do not. Discuss why the individuals look well dressed. What makes them look that way?

2. Do dressing make overs with before and after videotapes and pictures using clothing and accessories that are already in the client's wardrobe.

3. Have the client bring in soiled laundry and go to the community laundromat. Sort clothing according to color and water temperature, and follow directions on detergent box for correct usage. Insert correct coins and wash clothing.

4. Have a repair day where clients bring torn or buttonless clothing in to learn how to mend it.

5. Discuss what appropriate clothing to wear for occasion and weather (use pictures and magazine photos).

6. Discuss clothing according to matching color, texture, and pattern. Using cloth samples, coordinate an outfit.

7. Discuss proper fit, and the problems with clothing that is too large or too small.

8. Provide the opportunity for the client to look in a full length mirror at his back, front, and side views to determine if clothing is fitted correctly.

9. Identify proper wearing schedule for undergarments and clothing to ensure cleanliness.

10. Provide a check-off sheet so the client has a visual reminder to change clothing.

11. Practice reading clothing care tags on garments for cleaning and purchasing choices.

12. Compare the costs of dry cleaning a garment to washing a garment at the laundromat.

13. Discuss the differences in fabrics and what will have to be ironed versus permanent press. Discuss fabrics according to longevity and care.

14. Research newspapers and store flyers for the best values in clothing purchases such as jeans, socks, shoes, etc.

15. Discuss the pros and cons of following clothing fads versus purchasing more traditional clothing.

16. Discuss creative ways of finding inexpensive clothing (garage sales, thrift shops, Goodwill stores).

17. Discuss ways of hand-washing undergarments and delicate fabrics to save money at the laundromat.

18. Conduct a sewing group with an end goal of making an outfit. Discuss figure flaws and how to hide them, such as large stomach, wide hips, large thighs, etc.

19. Discuss different community resources that will provide free laundry soap to wash clothes.

20. Discuss attractive ways of wearing jewelry and accessories. Use pictures from magazines to identify ways of wearing scarves, hats, and jewelry.

# Chapter 7

# Grooming and Personal Hygiene

The purpose of this chapter is to list behavioral objectives according to the category of grooming and personal hygiene. Grooming activities involve obtaining and using supplies to shave; apply and remove cosmetics; wash, comb, style, and brush hair; care for nails; and care for skin. Personal hygiene activities involve obtaining and using supplies that promote cleanliness, such as bathing, applying deodorant, mouth care, and menses care. Additional areas addressed are safe use of grooming appliances and eyeglass care.

Grooming and personal hygiene is an area of independent living skills that is based on values and social/cultural influences. Cleanliness for one person may not be the same for another, when determining the frequency for taking a shower or shampooing hair. Lack of personal hygiene may be the first sign of emotional problems. Ambivalence toward grooming is a difficult attitude to overcome for some individuals who are experiencing mental illness. Some individuals' personal hygiene improves when they are taking psychotropic medications or not experiencing psychotic episodes. Since personal values, judgments, and opinions are so prevalent in determining correct personal hygiene routines, the health care professional must determine a minimum standard for socially appropriate grooming.

Personal cleanliness and appearance is important when trying to secure social contacts and employment. A person who emits strong body odor or appears disheveled will be ostracized by the community at large. It is important to assist clients in determining a thorough personal hygiene routine, in addition to emphasizing the consequences for not assuming responsibility for grooming. Areas to be addressed are sequences of bathing, hair care, shaving, toothbrushing, nail care, menses care, safe use of electrical grooming appliances, application of cosmetics, and eyeglass care.

*Table 7-1*

| Grooming and Hygiene | Objective | | | |
|---|---|---|---|---|
| **Behavioral Task** | **Condition of Performance** | **Frequency or Duration** | **Criteria for Moving to the Next Level of Performance** | **Time Frame** |
| **Personal Hygiene** | | | | |
| **Bathing.** The client will: | -with maximum physical guidance | 1 time per minute | 1 out of 3 times | by: (1 hour) |
| Identify correct frequency for bathing (sponge bath, shower, tub, or wash at sink). | -with moderate physical guidance | 3 times per minute | 3 out of 6 times | by: (6 hours) |
| Demonstrate an awareness of self body odor. | -with minimal physical guidance | 5 times per minute | __ out of __ times | by: (__ hours) |
| | -with ___% physical guidance | 1 time per hour | 4 consecutive trials out of 8 | by: (1 day) |
| Demonstrate awareness of when bathing is required. | -with tactile cues | 3 times per hour | 12 consecutive trials out of 15 | by: (3 days) |
| | -with a demonstration | 5 times per hour | __ consecutive trials out of __ | by: (__ days) |
| Demonstrate awareness of correct body parts to wash at the sink. | -with less than 5 verbal prompts | 6 consecutive times per hour | 20% of the time | by: (1 week) |
| Demonstrate awareness of correct body parts to wash in the tub/shower. | -with less than 3 verbal prompts | 2 times per day | 50% of the time | by: (3 weeks) |
| | -with 1 verbal prompt | 3 times per day | ___% of the time | by: (1 month) |
| Set up supplies for tub/shower (bath mat, towel, shampoo, razor, washcloth, soap). | -with maximum assistance | 6 times per day | | by: (6 weeks) |
| | -with moderate assistance | 1 time per week | | by: (8 weeks) |
| Place bathing supplies within reach of tub, shower, or sink prior to bathing (towel, washcloth, soap, razor, deodorant). | -with minimum assistance | 3 times per week | | by: (3 months) |
| | -with ___% assistance | 8 times per week | | by: (__ months) |
| Regulate water temperature before bathing. | -in the therapy setting | 1 time per month | | |
| Initiate bathing (sponge bath, shower, tub, or wash at sink). | -in the home setting | 3 times per month | | |
| Lather and wash total body during tub/shower. | -independently | 6 times per month | | |
| | -safely | | | |
| Rinse body during tub/shower. | | | | |

Table 7-1 (Continued)

| Grooming and Hygiene | Objective | | | |
|---|---|---|---|---|
| **Behavioral Task** | **Condition of Performance** | **Frequency or Duration** | **Criteria for Moving to the Next Level of Performance** | **Time Frame** |
| Dry body thoroughly following tub/shower. | -with maximum physical guidance | 1 time per minute | 1 out of 3 times | by: (1 hour) |
| Demonstrate awareness of cleanliness. | -with moderate physical guidance | 3 times per minute | 3 out of 6 times | by: (6 hours) |
|  | -with minimal physical guidance | 5 times per minute | __ out of __ times | by: (__ hours) |
| Demonstrate awareness of when to apply deodorant. | -with ___% physical guidance | 1 time per hour | 4 consecutive trials out of 8 | by: (1 day) |
| Initiate applying deodorant following bathing. | -with tactile cues | 3 times per hour | 12 consecutive trials out of 15 | by: (3 days) |
| Put away bathing supplies following activity. | -with a demonstration | 5 times per hour | __ consecutive trials out of __ | by: (__ days) |
| Hang bath mat and towels to dry after bathing. | -with less than 5 verbal prompts | 6 consecutive times per hour | 20% of the time | by: (1 week) |
|  | -with less than 3 verbal prompts | 2 times per day | 50% of the time | by: (3 weeks) |
| Put soiled linen and clothing in hamper following bathing. | -with 1 verbal prompt | 3 times per day | ___% of the time | by: (1 month) |
| Demonstrate knowledge of when to wash hands (before meals, when they are dirty, following toileting). | -with maximum assistance | 6 times per day | | by: (6 weeks) |
|  | -with moderate assistance | 1 time per week | | by: (8 weeks) |
| Initiate hand washing prior to meals. | -with minimum assistance | 3 times per week | | by: (3 months) |
| Initiate hand washing following toileting. | -with ___% assistance | 8 times per week | | by: (__ months) |
| Wash hands as needed. | -in the therapy setting | 1 time per month | | |
| **Mouth Care.** The client will: | -in the home setting | 3 times per month | | |
| Demonstrate awareness of correct frequency of toothbrushing (following meals, bedtime). | -independently | 6 times per month | | |
| Initiate toothbrushing. | | | | |

© SLACK Inc.

37

*Table 7-1 (Continued)*

| Grooming and Hygiene | Objective | | | |
|---|---|---|---|---|
| **Behavioral Task** | **Condition of Performance** | **Frequency or Duration** | **Criteria for Moving to the Next Level of Performance** | **Time Frame** |
| Apply toothpaste to brush prior to brushing teeth. | -with maximum physical guidance | 1 time per minute | 1 out of 3 times | by: (1 hour) |
| | -with moderate physical guidance | 3 times per minute | 3 out of 6 times | by: (6 hours) |
| Brush all surfaces of the teeth (anterior, posterior, lateral surfaces, and tongue). | -with minimal physical guidance | 5 times per minute | __ out of __ times | by: (__ hours) |
| Floss teeth. | -with ___% physical guidance | 1 time per hour | 4 consecutive trials out of 8 | by: (1 day) |
| Rinse mouth following toothbrushing. | -with tactile cues | 3 times per hour | 12 consecutive trials out of 15 | by: (3 days) |
| Rinse toothbrush following toothbrushing. | -with a demonstration | 5 times per hour | __ consecutive trials out of __ | by: (__ days) |
| Use mouth wash as needed. | -with less than 5 verbal prompts | 6 consecutive times per hour | 20% of the time | by: (1 week) |
| Initiate dental care. | -with less than 3 verbal prompts | 2 times per day | 50% of the time | by: (3 weeks) |
| Identify frequency of cleaning dentures (following meals, bedtime). | -with 1 verbal prompt | 3 times per day | ___% of the time | by: (1 month) |
| Remove dentures and place in denture cup. | -with maximum assistance | 6 times per day | | by: (6 weeks) |
| Brush gums before cleaning dentures. | -with moderate assistance | 1 time per week | | by: (8 weeks) |
| Brush dentures thoroughly. | -with minimum assistance | 3 times per week | | by: (3 months) |
| | -with ___% assistance | 8 times per week | | by: (__ months) |
| Place dentures correctly in mouth following brushing. | -in the therapy setting | 1 time per month | | |
| **Menses Care.** The client will: | -in the home setting | 3 times per month | | |
| Demonstrate awareness of start of menstrual flow. | -independently | 6 times per month | | |
| Demonstrate awareness of use of sanitary napkins/tampons. | | | | |

*Table 7-1 (Continued)*

| Grooming and Hygiene | | Objective | | |
|---|---|---|---|---|
| **Behavioral Task** | **Condition of Performance** | **Frequency or Duration** | **Criteria for Moving to the Next Level of Performance** | **Time Frame** |
| Change sanitary napkin/tampon when needed. | -with maximum physical guidance | 1 time per minute | 1 out of 3 times | by: (1 hour) |
| Dispose of sanitary napkin/tampon correctly. | -with moderate physical guidance | 3 times per minute | 3 out of 6 times | by: (6 hours) |
| Buy napkin/tampon from a machine. | -with minimal physical guidance | 5 times per minute | __ out of __ times | by: (__ hours) |
| Wash hands following handling of napkin/tampon | -with ___% physical guidance | 1 time per hour | 4 consecutive trials out of 8 | by: (1 day) |
| | -with tactile cues | 3 times per hour | 12 consecutive trials out of 15 | by: (3 days) |
| Cleanse self (genitals) following handling of napkin/tampon. | -with a demonstration | 5 times per hour | __ consecutive trials out of __ | by: (__ days) |
| Demonstrate an awareness of need for more frequent bathing during menses. | -with less than 5 verbal prompts | 6 consecutive times per hour | 20% of the time | by: (1 week) |
| | -with less than 3 verbal prompts | 2 times per day | 50% of the time | by: (3 weeks) |
| **Grooming** | -with 1 verbal prompt | 3 times per day | ___% of the time | by: (1 month) |
| **Hair Care.** The client will: | -with maximum assistance | 6 times per day | | by: (6 weeks) |
| Demonstrate awareness of when hair requires washing. | -with moderate assistance | 1 time per week | | by: (8 weeks) |
| Set up supplies for shampooing in the sink (towel, shampoo, conditioner). | -with minimum assistance | 3 times per week | | by: (3 months) |
| Initiate hair washing. | -with ___% assistance | 8 times per week | | by: (__ months) |
| Lather hair thoroughly during shampoo. | -in the therapy setting | 1 time per month | | |
| Regulate water temperature before rinsing at the sink. | -in the home setting | 3 times per month | | |
| Rinse hair thoroughly following shampoo. | -independently | 6 times per month | | |
| Apply conditioner following rinsing. | | | | |

© SLACK Inc.

39

*Table 7-1 (Continued)*

| Grooming and Hygiene | Objective | | | |
|---|---|---|---|---|
| **Behavioral Task** | **Condition of Performance** | **Frequency or Duration** | **Criteria for Moving to the Next Level of Performance** | **Time Frame** |
| Rinse hair following conditioning. | -with maximum physical guidance | 1 time per minute | 1 out of 3 times | by: (1 hour) |
| Demonstrate awareness of when to comb/ brush hair. | -with moderate physical guidance | 3 times per minute | 3 out of 6 times | by: (6 hours) |
| Initiate combing or brushing hair when needed. | -with minimal physical guidance | 5 times per minute | __ out of __ times | by: (__ hours) |
| | -with ___% physical guidance | 1 time per hour | 4 consecutive trials out of 8 | by: (1 day) |
| Use brush or comb to untangle hair when necessary. | -with tactile cues | 3 times per hour | 12 consecutive trials out of 15 | by: (3 days) |
| Identify when a haircut is required. | -with a demonstration | 5 times per hour | __ consecutive trials out of __ | by: (__ days) |
| Make arrangements to receive a haircut. | -with less than 5 verbal prompts | 6 consecutive times per hour | 20% of the time | by: (1 week) |
| Demonstrate an awareness of an attractive hairstyle on self. | -with less than 3 verbal prompts | 2 times per day | 50% of the time | by: (3 weeks) |
| | -with 1 verbal prompt | 3 times per day | ___% of the time | by: (1 month) |
| Initiate completion of an attractive hairstyle on self. | -with maximum assistance | 6 times per day | | by: (6 weeks) |
| | -with moderate assistance | 1 time per week | | by: (8 weeks) |
| Use electric hairstyling equipment (curling iron, electric rollers, blow dryer) in a safe manner. | -with minimum assistance | 3 times per week | | by: (3 months) |
| | -with ___% assistance | 8 times per week | | by: (__ months) |
| Set hair in rollers as needed. | -in the therapy setting | 1 time per month | | |
| Use hair spray in a safe manner. | -in the home setting | 3 times per month | | |
| **Nail Care.** The client will: | -independently | 6 times per month | | |
| Demonstrate awareness of when nails require cleaning. | | | | |
| Initiate nail cleaning. | | | | |

*Table 7-1 (Continued)*

| Grooming and Hygiene | Objective | | | |
|---|---|---|---|---|
| **Behavioral Task** | **Condition of Performance** | **Frequency or Duration** | **Criteria for Moving to the Next Level of Performance** | **Time Frame** |
| Demonstrate awareness of when to trim nails. | -with maximum physical guidance | 1 time per minute | 1 out of 3 times | by: (1 hour) |
| Initiate nail trimming on hands and feet. | -with moderate physical guidance | 3 times per minute | 3 out of 6 times | by: (6 hours) |
| Polish nails in a correct and attractive manner. | -with minimal physical guidance | 5 times per minute | __ out of __ times | by: (__ hours) |
| | -with ___% physical guidance | 1 time per hour | 4 consecutive trials out of 8 | by: (1 day) |
| Remove nail polish when it becomes chipped or cracked. | -with tactile cues | 3 times per hour | 12 consecutive trials out of 15 | by: (3 days) |
| **Shaving.** The client will: | -with a demonstration | 5 times per hour | __ consecutive trials out of __ | by: (__ days) |
| Demonstrate awareness of when to shave. | -with less than 5 verbal prompts | 6 consecutive times per hour | 20% of the time | by: (1 week) |
| Obtain shaving supplies including shaving cream, towel, and razor. | -with less than 3 verbal prompts | 2 times per day | 50% of the time | by: (3 weeks) |
| | -with 1 verbal prompt | 3 times per day | ___% of the time | by: (1 month) |
| Use a razor (straight-edge) safely. | -with maximum assistance | 6 times per day | | by: (6 weeks) |
| Wet area of face to be shaved. | -with moderate assistance | 1 time per week | | by: (8 weeks) |
| Apply shaving cream or skin softener prior to shaving. | -with minimum assistance | 3 times per week | | by: (3 months) |
| Shave both cheeks (downward motion). | -with ___% assistance | 8 times per week | | by: (__ months) |
| Rinse blade as necessary. | -in the therapy setting | 1 time per month | | |
| Shave under nose (downward motion). | -in the home setting | 3 times per month | | |
| Shave neck. | -independently | 6 times per month | | |
| Inspect face in mirror to determine if all areas have been shaved. | | | | |

© SLACK Inc.

*Table 7-1 (Continued)*

| *Grooming and Hygiene* | **Objective** | | | |
|---|---|---|---|---|
| **Behavioral Task** | **Condition of Performance** | **Frequency or Duration** | **Criteria for Moving to the Next Level of Performance** | **Time Frame** |
| Rinse off excess lather from face and dry face. | -with maximum physical guidance | 1 time per minute | 1 out of 3 times | by: (1 hour) |
| Clean and dry razor following use. | -with moderate physical guidance | 3 times per minute | 3 out of 6 times | by: (6 hours) |
| Change blade in razor if dull, or indicate if it is dull. | -with minimal physical guidance | 5 times per minute | __ out of __ times | by: (__ hours) |
| | -with ___% physical guidance | 1 time per hour | 4 consecutive trials out of 8 | by: (1 day) |
| Use an electric razor safely. | -with tactile cues | 3 times per hour | 12 consecutive trials out of 15 | by: (3 days) |
| Plug in razor. | -with a demonstration | 5 times per hour | __ consecutive trials out of __ | by: (__ days) |
| Shave both cheeks using a circular motion. | -with less than 5 verbal prompts | 6 consecutive times per hour | 20% of the time | by: (1 week) |
| Shut off electric razor following use. | -with less than 3 verbal prompts | 2 times per day | 50% of the time | by: (3 weeks) |
| Clean electric razor following use. | -with 1 verbal prompt | 3 times per day | ___% of the time | by: (1 month) |
| Put shaving supplies away following use. | -with maximum assistance | 6 times per day | | by: (6 weeks) |
| Trim mustache and beard as needed. | -with moderate assistance | 1 time per week | | by: (8 weeks) |
| **Skin Care.** The client will: | -with minimum assistance | 3 times per week | | by: (3 months) |
| Protect skin from the sun by using a sunscreen. | -with ___% assistance | 8 times per week | | by: (__ months) |
| Use moisturizer to prevent dry skin when necessary. | -in the therapy setting | 1 time per month | | |
| | -in the home setting | 3 times per month | | |
| Protect lips by using lip balm during cold weather. | -independently | 6 times per month | | |
| Apply moisturizer following shaving as needed. | | | | |

*Table 7-1 (Continued)*

| Grooming and Hygiene | Objective | | | |
|---|---|---|---|---|
| **Behavioral Task** | **Condition of Performance** | **Frequency or Duration** | **Criteria for Moving to the Next Level of Performance** | **Time Frame** |
| Select cosmetics according to skin type (dry, oily). | -with maximum physical guidance | 1 time per minute | 1 out of 3 times | by: (1 hour) |
| | -with moderate physical guidance | 3 times per minute | 3 out of 6 times | by: (6 hours) |
| **Nose Care.** The client will: | -with minimal physical guidance | 5 times per minute | __ out of __ times | by: (__ hours) |
| Trim nose hair as needed. | -with ___% physical guidance | 1 time per hour | 4 consecutive trials out of 8 | by: (1 day) |
| Blow nose and clear nasal area as needed. | -with tactile cues | 3 times per hour | 12 consecutive trials out of 15 | by: (3 days) |
| Use a tissue or cloth handkerchief to blow nose when needed. | -with a demonstration | 5 times per hour | __ consecutive trials out of __ | by: (__ days) |
| **Eye Care.** The client will: | -with less than 5 verbal prompts | 6 consecutive times per hour | 20% of the time | by: (1 week) |
| Clean corners of eyes as needed. | -with less than 3 verbal prompts | 2 times per day | 50% of the time | by: (3 weeks) |
| Demonstrate an awareness of when eyeglasses are dirty. | -with 1 verbal prompt | 3 times per day | ___% of the time | by: (1 month) |
| | -with maximum assistance | 6 times per day | | by: (6 weeks) |
| Initiate cleaning of eyeglasses when dirty. | -with moderate assistance | 1 time per week | | by: (8 weeks) |
| Take eyeglasses to be repaired or adjusted when needed. | -with minimum assistance | 3 times per week | | by: (3 months) |
| **Ear Care.** The client will: | -with ___% assistance | 8 times per week | | by: (__ months) |
| Clean ears as needed. | -in the therapy setting | 1 time per month | | |
| Clean pierced earlobes with alcohol as needed. | -in the home setting | 3 times per month | | |
| Clean pierced earrings with alcohol prior to inserting as needed. | -independently | 6 times per month | | |

© SLACK Inc.

*Table 7-1 (Continued)*

| Grooming and Hygiene | | Objective | | |
|---|---|---|---|---|

| Behavioral Task | Condition of Performance | Frequency or Duration | Criteria for Moving to the Next Level of Performance | Time Frame |
|---|---|---|---|---|
| **Cosmetics.** The client will: | | | | |
| Read labels on cosmetics for appropriate and safe use. | -with maximum physical guidance | 1 time per minute | 1 out of 3 times | by: (1 hour) |
| | -with moderate physical guidance | 3 times per minute | 3 out of 6 times | by: (6 hours) |
| Apply makeup in a correct and attractive manner. | -with minimal physical guidance | 5 times per minute | __ out of __ times | by: (__ hours) |
| Remove makeup using appropriate cleanser. | -with ___% physical guidance | 1 time per hour | 4 consecutive trials out of 8 | by: (1 day) |
| Use appropriate amount of cologne or perfume. | -with tactile cues | 3 times per hour | 12 consecutive trials out of 15 | by: (3 days) |
| | -with a demonstration | 5 times per hour | __ consecutive trials out of __ | by: (__ days) |
| **Maintenance of Grooming Supplies** The client will: | -with less than 5 verbal prompts | 6 consecutive times per hour | 20% of the time | by: (1 week) |
| Replace supplies as needed. | -with less than 3 verbal prompts | 2 times per day | 50% of the time | by: (3 weeks) |
| Make a list of grooming supplies as needed. | -with 1 verbal prompt | 3 times per day | ___% of the time | by: (1 month) |
| Purchase grooming products as needed (shampoo, soap, cosmetics). | -with maximum assistance | 6 times per day | | by: (6 weeks) |
| | -with moderate assistance | 1 time per week | | by: (8 weeks) |
| Ask supportive other to purchase grooming supplies for them. | -with minimum assistance | 3 times per week | | by: (3 months) |
| | -with ___% assistance | 8 times per week | | by: (__ months) |
| | -in the therapy setting | 1 time per month | | |
| | -in the home setting | 3 times per month | | |
| | -independently | 6 times per month | | |

## Therapeutic Suggestions

1. Develop grooming routine charts so the client can check off each task in his/her morning personal hygiene routine that has been completed, repeating the process in the evening (pictorial, writing, or both).

2. Have the client put together a grooming kit in a zip lock bag. Make a list of the items that are in the kit so that they can be easily replaced by the client when they are gone. The grooming kit would also help prompt the client to complete a hygiene routine because all items in the kit would be used on a daily basis.

3. Discuss the consequences of not bathing routinely or following good personal hygiene routines (impact on others' perception of us, impact on self).

4. Do makeovers with change of hairstyle, makeup, and nails. Take before and after pictures or videotapes and discuss the changes with the client.

5. Have the client look at magazine pictures to get tips on hairstyles and application of cosmetics.

6. Show clients pictures of people in various stages of grooming, from disheveled to meticulous, and have them discriminate what is appropriate and what isn't.

7. Show a variety of grooming products (group or individual) and discuss use, cost, and where they can be purchased.

8. Demonstrate correct way to shave and apply deodorant, makeup, nail polish, and hair spray.

9. Have clients identify the correct supplies needed for grooming routines.

10. Have clients go over the purpose of cleanliness, hygiene, and grooming.

11. Have the clients perform a facial on themselves.

12. Demonstrate how to give a manicure and have clients give themselves one.

13. Go on a shopping trip to purchase grooming supplies. Compare brand names and prices for best value.

14. Have the client pick out a hairstyle from a magazine and make an appointment with a hairdresser.

15. Invite a Dental Hygienist to your group to demonstrate correct brushing and flossing, and the importance of good mouth care.

16. Invite a cosmetologist to come to your group and demonstrate correct application of makeup.

17. Demonstrate grooming appliances such as electric rollers, curling irons, and razors. Talk about price and safe use of these appliances.

18. Bring a variety of perfume or cologne samples to the group. Have the clients identify which smells they prefer and which ones they do not prefer. Discuss the importance of smell and its effect on others.

19. Have each client make a list of grooming supplies used throughout the week. Have them identify how much each item costs and how to obtain the items on a limited income. Discuss the need to prioritize (for example, purchasing soap may be more important than buying lipstick).

20. Discuss health-related issues regarding poor personal hygiene (disease, infection, gum disease, infestation, and skin and hair conditions); its effect on others.

# Chapter 8

# Household Management

The purpose of this chapter is to identify skills needed to maintain a household. Independent living is a major standard of success in rehabilitating persons with mental illnesses. Independent management of a personal residence encompasses all areas of independent living with the exception of securing a job.

Areas included in this chapter are how to select appropriate and affordable housing; cleaning, maintenance, and minor household repairs; pet and plant care; and making a residence safe for children. The reader will find that some skill areas typically found under household management are found in other chapters in this text, or are identified in their own chapters. Examples are meal preparation and cleanup which are found in Chapter 5, Food Consumption Activities; clothing care is found in Chapter 6, Dressing and Clothing Care; financial considerations are found in Chapter 11, Money Management; and household safety is found in Chapter 14, Life Safety Skills.

*Table 8-1*

| Household Management | | Objective | | |
|---|---|---|---|---|
| **Behavioral Task** | **Condition of Performance** | **Frequency or Duration** | **Criteria for Moving to the Next Level of Performance** | **Time Frame** |
| **Selection of Housing.** The client will: | | | | |
| Identify available Adult Foster Care homes. | -with maximum physical guidance | 1 time per minute | 1 out of 3 times | by: (1 hour) |
| Find out requirements to reside in an Adult Foster Care home (no smoking, number of roommates, curfew). | -with moderate physical guidance | 3 times per minute | 3 out of 6 times | by: (6 hours) |
| | -with minimal physical guidance | 5 times per minute | __ out of __ times | by: (__ hours) |
| Identify preferred Adult Foster Care home to case manager. | -with ___% physical guidance | 1 time per hour | 4 consecutive trials out of 8 | by: (1 day) |
| Identify an affordable apartment. | -with tactile cues | 3 times per hour | 12 consecutive trials out of 15 | by: (3 days) |
| | -with a demonstration | 5 times per hour | __ consecutive trials out of __ | by: (__ days) |
| Identify an appropriate apartment by location. | -with less than 5 verbal prompts | 6 consecutive times per hour | 20% of the time | by: (1 week) |
| Identify an appropriate apartment by appearance. | -with less than 3 verbal prompts | 2 times per day | 50% of the time | by: (3 weeks) |
| | -with 1 verbal prompt | 3 times per day | ___% of the time | by: (1 month) |
| Assess individual requirements for housing (cost, location, comfort, space). | -with maximum assistance | 6 times per day | | by: (6 weeks) |
| Contact apartment landlords and ask for information about rentals. | -with moderate assistance | 1 time per week | | by: (8 weeks) |
| | -with minimum assistance | 3 times per week | | by: (3 months) |
| Contact a subsidized housing facility for information. | -with ___% assistance | 8 times per week | | by: (__ months) |
| Fill out an application for renting an apartment. | -in the therapy setting | 1 time per month | | |
| | -in the home setting | 3 times per month | | |
| Find out the costs of utilities, phone, garbage disposal, and any additional expenses for a rental unit. | -in a community setting | 6 times per month | | |
| | -independently | | | |

Table 8-1 (Continued)

| Household Management | Objective | | | |
|---|---|---|---|---|
| **Behavioral Task** | **Condition of Performance** | **Frequency or Duration** | **Criteria for Moving to the Next Level of Performance** | **Time Frame** |
| Select appropriate housing by evaluating cost, location, space, appearance, and comfort. | -with maximum physical guidance | 1 time per minute | 1 out of 3 times | by: (1 hour) |
| | -with moderate physical guidance | 3 times per minute | 3 out of 6 times | by: (6 hours) |
| **Maintenance of Personal Space.** The client will: | -with minimal physical guidance | 5 times per minute | __ out of __ times | by: (__ hours) |
| | -with ___% physical guidance | 1 time per hour | 4 consecutive trials out of 8 | by: (1 day) |
| Put personal belongings and clothing in proper place when not in use. | -with tactile cues | 3 times per hour | 12 consecutive trials out of 15 | by: (3 days) |
| Put miscellaneous items in correct place following use (magazines, papers, games). | -with a demonstration | 5 times per hour | __ consecutive trials out of __ | by: (__ days) |
| | -with less than 5 verbal prompts | 6 consecutive times per hour | 20% of the time | by: (1 week) |
| Ensure that clean clothing, towels, bed linens (1 set), are always available. | -with less than 3 verbal prompts | 2 times per day | 50% of the time | by: (3 weeks) |
| Clean counters and surfaces of appliances. | -with 1 verbal prompt | 3 times per day | ___% of the time | by: (1 month) |
| Identify when garbage needs to be taken out, and take it out. | -with maximum assistance | 6 times per day | | by: (6 weeks) |
| | -with moderate assistance | 1 time per week | | by: (8 weeks) |
| Identify when toilet paper needs to be replaced, and replace it. | -with minimum assistance | 3 times per week | | by: (3 months) |
| Identify when tissue needs to be replaced, and replace it. | -with ___% assistance | 8 times per week | | by: (__ months) |
| | -in the therapy setting | 1 time per month | | |
| Identify when soap needs to be replaced, and replace it. | -in the home setting | 3 times per month | | |
| Identify when toothpaste needs to be replaced, and replace it. | -independently | 6 times per month | | |
| Identify when toothbrush needs replacing, and replace it. | | | | |

*Table 8-1 (Continued)*

| Household Management | Objective | | | |
|---|---|---|---|---|
| **Behavioral Task** | **Condition of Performance** | **Frequency or Duration** | **Criteria for Moving to the Next Level of Performance** | **Time Frame** |
| Identify when cleaning supplies need to be replaced, and replace them. | -with maximum physical guidance | 1 time per minute | 1 out of 3 times | by: (1 hour) |
| | -with moderate physical guidance | 3 times per minute | 3 out of 6 times | by: (6 hours) |
| **Storage.** The client will: | -with minimal physical guidance | 5 times per minute | __ out of __ times | by: (__ hours) |
| Select and organize an area to store medications. | -with ___% physical guidance | 1 time per hour | 4 consecutive trials out of 8 | by: (1 day) |
| Select and organize an area to store cleaning supplies. | -with tactile cues | 3 times per hour | 12 consecutive trials out of 15 | by: (3 days) |
| | -with a demonstration | 5 times per hour | __ consecutive trials out of __ | by: (__ days) |
| Select and organize an area to store common household tools (hammer, screwdriver, wrench). | -with less than 5 verbal prompts | 6 consecutive times per hour | 20% of the time | by: (1 week) |
| | -with less than 3 verbal prompts | 2 times per day | 50% of the time | by: (3 weeks) |
| Select and organize an area to store linens (towels, sheets). | -with 1 verbal prompt | 3 times per day | ___% of the time | by: (1 month) |
| Select and organize an area to store grooming supplies. | -with maximum assistance | 6 times per day | | by: (6 weeks) |
| | -with moderate assistance | 1 time per week | | by: (8 weeks) |
| Select and organize appropriate areas to store clothing. | -with minimum assistance | 3 times per week | | by: (3 months) |
| Select and organize an area to store sewing supplies. | -with ___% assistance | 8 times per week | | by: (__ months) |
| | -in the therapy setting | 1 time per month | | |
| Select and organize an area for miscellaneous items (beverage cans, newspapers, magazines). | -in the home setting | 3 times per month | | |
| Select a person to store personal property if hospitalized. | -independently | 6 times per month | | |

© SLACK Inc.

*Table 8-1 (Continued)*

| Household Management | | Objective | | |
|---|---|---|---|---|
| **Behavioral Task** | **Condition of Performance** | **Frequency or Duration** | **Criteria for Moving to the Next Level of Performance** | **Time Frame** |
| **Vacuuming**. The client will: | | | | |
| Identify need for vacuuming. | -with maximum physical guidance | 1 time per minute | 1 out of 3 times | by: (1 hour) |
| Retrieve vacuum from storage space. | -with moderate physical guidance | 3 times per minute | 3 out of 6 times | by: (6 hours) |
| Put correct attachments on vacuum. | -with minimal physical guidance | 5 times per minute | __ out of __ times | by: (__ hours) |
| Plug vacuum into wall socket. | -with ___% physical guidance | 1 time per hour | 4 consecutive trials out of 8 | by: (1 day) |
| Clear all lightweight articles off rug (wastebaskets, papers). | -with tactile cues | 3 times per hour | 12 consecutive trials out of 15 | by: (3 days) |
| Turn vacuum on. | -with a demonstration | 5 times per hour | __ consecutive trials out of __ | by: (__ days) |
| Move lightweight furniture to vacuum under and behind. | -with less than 5 verbal prompts | 6 consecutive times per hour | 20% of the time | by: (1 week) |
| | -with less than 3 verbal prompts | 2 times per day | 50% of the time | by: (3 weeks) |
| Vacuum whole floor space. | -with 1 verbal prompt | 3 times per day | ___% of the time | by: (1 month) |
| Turn off vacuum following use. | -with maximum assistance | 6 times per day | | by: (6 weeks) |
| Replace articles and furniture removed for vacuuming. | -with moderate assistance | 1 time per week | | by: (8 weeks) |
| | -with minimum assistance | 3 times per week | | by: (3 months) |
| Put vacuum and attachments away following use. | -with ___% assistance | 8 times per week | | by: (__ months) |
| Identify need to change vacuum bag and replace when necessary. | -in the therapy setting | 1 time per month | | |
| | -in the home setting | 3 times per month | | |
| **Sweep with a Broom.** The client will: | -independently | 6 times per month | | |
| Identify when floor needs to be swept. | | | | |

*Table 8-1 (Continued)*

| Household Management | **Objective** | | | |
|---|---|---|---|---|
| **Behavioral Task** | **Condition of Performance** | **Frequency or Duration** | **Criteria for Moving to the Next Level of Performance** | **Time Frame** |
| Retrieve a broom. | -with maximum physical guidance | 1 time per minute | 1 out of 3 times | by: (1 hour) |
| Sweep all dust and food particles to one area. | -with moderate physical guidance | 3 times per minute | 3 out of 6 times | by: (6 hours) |
| Pick up dust pan and place on the floor next to the swept dirt. | -with minimal physical guidance | 5 times per minute | __ out of __ times | by: (__ hours) |
| | -with ___% physical guidance | 1 time per hour | 4 consecutive trials out of 8 | by: (1 day) |
| Sweep dirt into dust pan. | -with tactile cues | 3 times per hour | 12 consecutive trials out of 15 | by: (3 days) |
| Dump dust from dust pan into trash can. | -with a demonstration | 5 times per hour | __ consecutive trials out of __ | by: (__ days) |
| Put broom and dust pan away following use. | -with less than 5 verbal prompts | 6 consecutive times per hour | 20% of the time | by: (1 week) |
| **Dusting.** The client will: | -with less than 3 verbal prompts | 2 times per day | 50% of the time | by: (3 weeks) |
| Identify when furniture, decorative wall pictures, and TV screen needs to be dusted. | -with 1 verbal prompt | 3 times per day | ___% of the time | by: (1 month) |
| Obtain supplies for dusting (rags, polish, dust cloths). | -with maximum assistance | 6 times per day | | by: (6 weeks) |
| | -with moderate assistance | 1 time per week | | by: (8 weeks) |
| Read directions for use on polish or spray. | -with minimum assistance | 3 times per week | | by: (3 months) |
| Remove articles from surface of furniture needing to be dusted. | -with ___% assistance | 8 times per week | | by: (__ months) |
| Spray furniture surface with polish. | -in the therapy setting | 1 time per month | | |
| Wipe surface with dust cloth. | -in the home setting | 3 times per month | | |
| Put supplies away following use. | -independently | 6 times per month | | |
| **Mopping.** The client will: | | | | |
| Identify when the floor needs to be mopped. | | | | |

© SLACK Inc.

*Table 8-1 (Continued)*

| Household Management | Objective | | | |
|---|---|---|---|---|
| **Behavioral Task** | **Condition of Performance** | **Frequency or Duration** | **Criteria for Moving to the Next Level of Performance** | **Time Frame** |
| Obtain supplies needed for mopping the floor (mop, bucket, soap/cleaning agent). | -with maximum physical guidance | 1 time per minute | 1 out of 3 times | by: (1 hour) |
| | -with moderate physical guidance | 3 times per minute | 3 out of 6 times | by: (6 hours) |
| Clear all lightweight moveable objects off the floor. | -with minimal physical guidance | 5 times per minute | __ out of __ times | by: (__ hours) |
| Read instructions for cleaning agent prior to use. | -with ___% physical guidance | 1 time per hour | 4 consecutive trials out of 8 | by: (1 day) |
| | -with tactile cues | 3 times per hour | 12 consecutive trials out of 15 | by: (3 days) |
| Place correct amount of cleaning agent and water in mop bucket. | -with a demonstration | 5 times per hour | __ consecutive trials out of __ | by: (__ days) |
| Wet mop, squeezing excess amount of water out. | -with less than 5 verbal prompts | 6 consecutive times per hour | 20% of the time | by: (1 week) |
| | -with less than 3 verbal prompts | 2 times per day | 50% of the time | by: (3 weeks) |
| Systematically mop floor surface starting in one corner and moving toward the center of the floor. | -with 1 verbal prompt | 3 times per day | ___% of the time | by: (1 month) |
| | -with maximum assistance | 6 times per day | | by: (6 weeks) |
| Continue to wet and squeeze out the mop. | -with moderate assistance | 1 time per week | | by: (8 weeks) |
| Empty mop bucket in sink following use. | -with minimum assistance | 3 times per week | | by: (3 months) |
| Rinse bucket and mop following use. | -with ___% assistance | 8 times per week | | by: (__ months) |
| Put mop, bucket, and cleaning agent away following use. | -in the therapy setting | 1 time per month | | |
| Replace articles removed following mopping. | -in the home setting | 3 times per month | | |
| **Bathtub Cleaning.** The client will: | -independently | 6 times per month | | |
| Identify when bathtub needs to be cleaned. | | | | |

*Table 8-1 (Continued)*

| Household Management | Objective | | | |
|---|---|---|---|---|
| **Behavioral Task** | **Condition of Performance** | **Frequency or Duration** | **Criteria for Moving to the Next Level of Performance** | **Time Frame** |
| Obtain supplies needed to clean bathtub (sponge/rag, rubber gloves, cleaning agent). | -with maximum physical guidance | 1 time per minute | 1 out of 3 times | by: (1 hour) |
| | -with moderate physical guidance | 3 times per minute | 3 out of 6 times | by: (6 hours) |
| Turn on water to wet bathtub prior to cleaning. | -with minimal physical guidance | 5 times per minute | __ out of __ times | by: (__ hours) |
| Wet sponge/rag. | -with ___% physical guidance | 1 time per hour | 4 consecutive trials out of 8 | by: (1 day) |
| Read directions for using cleanser/soap prior to cleaning bathtub. | -with tactile cues | 3 times per hour | 12 consecutive trials out of 15 | by: (3 days) |
| Apply cleaning agent to bathtub surface. | -with a demonstration | 5 times per hour | __ consecutive trials out of __ | by: (__ days) |
| Rub all surfaces of the tub with the sponge. | -with less than 5 verbal prompts | 6 consecutive times per hour | 20% of the time | by: (1 week) |
| Rinse off cleaning agent with sponge and running water. | -with less than 3 verbal prompts | 2 times per day | 50% of the time | by: (3 weeks) |
| Wring out sponge. | -with 1 verbal prompt | 3 times per day | ___% of the time | by: (1 month) |
| Put all bathtub cleaning supplies away following use. | -with maximum assistance | 6 times per day | | by: (6 weeks) |
| | -with moderate assistance | 1 time per week | | by: (8 weeks) |
| Clean shower curtain and liner when needed. | -with minimum assistance | 3 times per week | | by: (3 months) |
| Replace shower curtain liner when needed. | -with ___% assistance | 8 times per week | | by: (__ months) |
| **Toilet Cleaning.** The client will: | -in the therapy setting | 1 time per month | | |
| Identify when toilet needs to be cleaned. | -in the home setting | 3 times per month | | |
| Obtain cleaning supplies for toilet (brush, sponge, cleaning agent). | -independently | 6 times per month | | |
| Wet sponge in sink and wring out. | | | | |

© SLACK Inc.

*Table 8-1 (Continued)*

| Household Management | Objective | | | |
|---|---|---|---|---|
| **Behavioral Task** | **Condition of Performance** | **Frequency or Duration** | **Criteria for Moving to the Next Level of Performance** | **Time Frame** |
| Apply cleaning agent to sponge or directly on toilet tank and lid. | -with maximum physical guidance | 1 time per minute | 1 out of 3 times | by: (1 hour) |
| Rub toilet tank and lid with sponge. | -with moderate physical guidance | 3 times per minute | 3 out of 6 times | by: (6 hours) |
| Apply cleaning agent to toilet seat, under lid, and outside of bowl. | -with minimal physical guidance | 5 times per minute | __ out of __ times | by: (__ hours) |
| | -with ___% physical guidance | 1 time per hour | 4 consecutive trials out of 8 | by: (1 day) |
| Wipe sponge on toilet seat, under lid, and outside of bowl. | -with tactile cues | 3 times per hour | 12 consecutive trials out of 15 | by: (3 days) |
| Rinse sponge and wring out. | -with a demonstration | 5 times per hour | __ consecutive trials out of __ | by: (__ days) |
| Put cleaning agent on inside of toilet bowl. | -with less than 5 verbal prompts | 6 consecutive times per hour | 20% of the time | by: (1 week) |
| Use scrub brush to cleanse inside of toilet bowl and under the upper lid. | -with less than 3 verbal prompts | 2 times per day | 50% of the time | by: (3 weeks) |
| | -with 1 verbal prompt | 3 times per day | ___% of the time | by: (1 month) |
| Flush toilet bowl following cleaning. | -with maximum assistance | 6 times per day | | by: (6 weeks) |
| Rinse scrub brush and sponge following use. | -with moderate assistance | 1 time per week | | by: (8 weeks) |
| Put toilet cleaning supplies away following use. | -with minimum assistance | 3 times per week | | by: (3 months) |
| **Wash Sink.** The client will: | -with ___% assistance | 8 times per week | | by: (__ months) |
| Obtain cleaning supplies for sink (sponge, cleanser). | -in the therapy setting | 1 time per month | | |
| Wet sink prior to cleaning. | -in the home setting | 3 times per month | | |
| Place appropriate amount of cleanser in sink bowl. | -independently | 6 times per month | | |
| Scrub inside and outside of sink bowl. | | | | |

*Table 8-1 (Continued)*

| Household Management | Objective | | | |
|---|---|---|---|---|
| **Behavioral Task** | **Condition of Performance** | **Frequency or Duration** | **Criteria for Moving to the Next Level of Performance** | **Time Frame** |
| Scrub counter surface surrounding sink bowl. | -with maximum physical guidance | 1 time per minute | 1 out of 3 times | by: (1 hour) |
| Scrub sink fixtures. | -with moderate physical guidance | 3 times per minute | 3 out of 6 times | by: (6 hours) |
| Remove and scrub all surfaces of sink traps. | -with minimal physical guidance | 5 times per minute | __ out of __ times | by: (__ hours) |
| Rinse sink, fixtures, and traps with sponge and running water. | -with ___% physical guidance | 1 time per hour | 4 consecutive trials out of 8 | by: (1 day) |
| Rinse sponge following use. | -with tactile cues | 3 times per hour | 12 consecutive trials out of 15 | by: (3 days) |
| | -with a demonstration | 5 times per hour | __ consecutive trials out of __ | by: (__ days) |
| Put all sink cleaning supplies away following use. | -with less than 5 verbal prompts | 6 consecutive times per hour | 20% of the time | by: (1 week) |
| Turn on garbage disposal and run cold water for several seconds following cleaning of sink. | -with less than 3 verbal prompts | 2 times per day | 50% of the time | by: (3 weeks) |
| | -with 1 verbal prompt | 3 times per day | ___% of the time | by: (1 month) |
| **Cleaning and Organizing Cupboards.** The client will: | -with maximum assistance | 6 times per day | | by: (6 weeks) |
| | -with moderate assistance | 1 time per week | | by: (8 weeks) |
| Identify when cupboard needs to be cleaned. | -with minimum assistance | 3 times per week | | by: (3 months) |
| Remove all articles from the cupboard. | -with ___% assistance | 8 times per week | | by: (__ months) |
| Wipe cupboard shelves, sides, and top with a damp sponge. | -in the therapy setting | 1 time per month | | |
| Wipe off the front, tops, and sides of cupboard doors. | -in the home setting | 3 times per month | | |
| | -independently | 6 times per month | | |
| Throw away old food and empty containers. | | | | |
| Replace all items in cupboard so they are visible. | | | | |

*Table 8-1 (Continued)*

| Household Management | Objective | | | |
|---|---|---|---|---|
| **Behavioral Task** | **Condition of Performance** | **Frequency or Duration** | **Criteria for Moving to the Next Level of Performance** | **Time Frame** |
| Store all items in cupboards according to use (cooking supplies near stove, supplies used with water by sink). | -with maximum physical guidance | 1 time per minute | 1 out of 3 times | by: (1 hour) |
| | -with moderate physical guidance | 3 times per minute | 3 out of 6 times | by: (6 hours) |
| **Cleaning a Refrigerator.** The client will: | -with minimal physical guidance | 5 times per minute | __ out of __ times | by: (__ hours) |
| Identify when refrigerator needs to be cleaned. | -with ___% physical guidance | 1 time per hour | 4 consecutive trials out of 8 | by: (1 day) |
| Obtain supplies needed to clean refrigerator (sponge, soapy water). | -with tactile cues | 3 times per hour | 12 consecutive trials out of 15 | by: (3 days) |
| Remove all food items from the refrigerator. | -with a demonstration | 5 times per hour | __ consecutive trials out of __ | by: (__ days) |
| Dispose of spoiled or old food. | -with less than 5 verbal prompts | 6 consecutive times per hour | 20% of the time | by: (1 week) |
| Throw away empty containers from refrigerator. | -with less than 3 verbal prompts | 2 times per day | 50% of the time | by: (3 weeks) |
| | -with 1 verbal prompt | 3 times per day | ___% of the time | by: (1 month) |
| Wipe refrigerator shelves with damp sponge. | -with maximum assistance | 6 times per day | | by: (6 weeks) |
| Wipe the walls of the refrigerator with a damp sponge. | -with moderate assistance | 1 time per week | | by: (8 weeks) |
| | -with minimum assistance | 3 times per week | | by: (3 months) |
| Replace remaining items in refrigerator. | -with ___% assistance | 8 times per week | | by: (__ months) |
| Clean outside of refrigerator. | -in the therapy setting | 1 time per month | | |
| Put away supplies used to clean refrigerator. | -in the home setting | 3 times per month | | |
| **Defrosting a Refrigerator.** The client will: | -independently | 6 times per month | | |
| Identify when refrigerator needs defrosting. | | | | |
| Put pot of water on the stove to boil. | | | | |

© SLACK Inc.

Table 8-1 (Continued)

| Household Management | | Objective | | |
|---|---|---|---|---|
| **Behavioral Task** | **Condition of Performance** | **Frequency or Duration** | **Criteria for Moving to the Next Level of Performance** | **Time Frame** |
| Turn refrigerator to "off" or "defrost." | -with maximum physical guidance | 1 time per minute | 1 out of 3 times | by: (1 hour) |
| Place towel on floor at base of refrigerator. | -with moderate physical guidance | 3 times per minute | 3 out of 6 times | by: (6 hours) |
| Take all food items out of refrigerator and freezer. | -with minimal physical guidance | 5 times per minute | __ out of __ times | by: (__ hours) |
| Place frozen food in sink while defrosting. | -with ___% physical guidance | 1 time per hour | 4 consecutive trials out of 8 | by: (1 day) |
| Place other food on counter while defrosting. | -with tactile cues | 3 times per hour | 12 consecutive trials out of 15 | by: (3 days) |
| Place pot of water in refrigerator. | -with a demonstration | 5 times per hour | __ consecutive trials out of __ | by: (__ days) |
| Empty freezer tray in sink when necessary. | -with less than 5 verbal prompts | 6 consecutive times per hour | 20% of the time | by: (1 week) |
| Empty ice into sink if necessary. | -with less than 3 verbal prompts | 2 times per day | 50% of the time | by: (3 weeks) |
| Reheat pot of water as needed. | -with 1 verbal prompt | 3 times per day | ___% of the time | by: (1 month) |
| Empty pot of water into sink following use. | -with maximum assistance | 6 times per day | | by: (6 weeks) |
| Dry out inside of refrigerator with towel following defrosting. | -with moderate assistance | 1 time per week | | by: (8 weeks) |
| Replace food items in refrigerator and freezer. | -with minimum assistance | 3 times per week | | by: (3 months) |
| | -with ___% assistance | 8 times per week | | by: (__ months) |
| Turn refrigerator back on. | -in the therapy setting | 1 time per month | | |
| **Cleaning an Oven.** The client will: | -in the home setting | 3 times per month | | |
| Identify when the oven needs to be cleaned. | -independently | 6 times per month | | |
| Obtain supplies for cleaning the oven (newspapers, oven cleaner, scrub brush, sponge). | -safely | | | |

*Table 8-1 (Continued)*

| Household Management | Objective | | | |
|---|---|---|---|---|
| **Behavioral Task** | **Condition of Performance** | **Frequency or Duration** | **Criteria for Moving to the Next Level of Performance** | **Time Frame** |
| Place newspapers on the floor at the base of the oven. | -with maximum physical guidance | 1 time per minute | 1 out of 3 times | by: (1 hour) |
| Carefully read oven cleaner instructions. | -with moderate physical guidance | 3 times per minute | 3 out of 6 times | by: (6 hours) |
| Follow application and heating instructions for oven cleaner. | -with minimal physical guidance | 5 times per minute | __ out of __ times | by: (__ hours) |
| | -with ___% physical guidance | 1 time per hour | 4 consecutive trials out of 8 | by: (1 day) |
| Wipe walls and floor of oven following appropriate application of oven cleaner. | -with tactile cues | 3 times per hour | 12 consecutive trials out of 15 | by: (3 days) |
| Scrub stubborn spots with brush if necessary. | -with a demonstration | 5 times per hour | __ consecutive trials out of __ | by: (__ days) |
| | -with less than 5 verbal prompts | 6 consecutive times per hour | 20% of the time | by: (1 week) |
| Thoroughly rinse out inside of oven with sponge and wipe dry. | -with less than 3 verbal prompts | 2 times per day | 50% of the time | by: (3 weeks) |
| Replace oven racks, if appropriate, following cleaning. | -with 1 verbal prompt | 3 times per day | ___% of the time | by: (1 month) |
| | -with maximum assistance | 6 times per day | | by: (6 weeks) |
| **Bed Making.** The client will: | -with moderate assistance | 1 time per week | | by: (8 weeks) |
| Identify when bed needs to be made. | -with minimum assistance | 3 times per week | | by: (3 months) |
| Remove pillow from bed. | -with ___% assistance | 8 times per week | | by: (__ months) |
| Smooth bottom sheet with hand. | -in the therapy setting | 1 time per month | | |
| Pull top sheet to top of mattress. | -in the home setting | 3 times per month | | |
| Smooth out wrinkles on top sheet. | -independently | 6 times per month | | |
| Pull blanket to top of mattress. | -safely | | | |
| Smooth out wrinkles in blanket. | | | | |

*Table 8-1 (Continued)*

| Household Management | **Objective** | | | |
|---|---|---|---|---|
| **Behavioral Task** | **Condition of Performance** | **Frequency or Duration** | **Criteria for Moving to the Next Level of Performance** | **Time Frame** |
| Tuck blanket and top sheet into bottom of mattress if necessary. | -with maximum physical guidance | 1 time per minute | 1 out of 3 times | by: (1 hour) |
| Replace pillow on bed. | -with moderate physical guidance | 3 times per minute | 3 out of 6 times | by: (6 hours) |
| Pull bedspread over bed. | -with minimal physical guidance | 5 times per minute | ___ out of ___ times | by: (___ hours) |
| Straighten bedspread and smooth out wrinkles. | -with ___% physical guidance | 1 time per hour | 4 consecutive trials out of 8 | by: (1 day) |
| | -with tactile cues | 3 times per hour | 12 consecutive trials out of 15 | by: (3 days) |
| Tuck bedspread under pillow to form crease. | -with a demonstration | 5 times per hour | ___ consecutive trials out of ___ | by: (___ days) |
| **Changing Bed Linen.** The client will: | -with less than 5 verbal prompts | 6 consecutive times per hour | 20% of the time | by: (1 week) |
| Identify when bed linen needs to be changed. | -with less than 3 verbal prompts | 2 times per day | 50% of the time | by: (3 weeks) |
| Strip soiled linens and blankets from bed. | -with 1 verbal prompt | 3 times per day | ___% of the time | by: (1 month) |
| Place soiled linens in laundry. | -with maximum assistance | 6 times per day | | by: (6 weeks) |
| Obtain a clean fitted sheet, top sheet, and pillow case. | -with moderate assistance | 1 time per week | | by: (8 weeks) |
| | -with minimum assistance | 3 times per week | | by: (3 months) |
| Put clean linens on bed. | -with ___% assistance | 8 times per week | | by: (___ months) |
| **Washing Windows and Mirrors.** The client will: | -in the therapy setting | 1 time per month | | |
| | -in the home setting | 3 times per month | | |
| Identify when windows and mirrors need to be washed. | -independently | 6 times per month | | |
| Obtain supplies for washing windows and mirrors (ladder, rags, cleanser, newspaper). | | | | |
| Safely set up a stool or ladder to stand on. | | | | |

*Table 8-1 (Continued)*

| Household Management | | Objective | | |
|---|---|---|---|---|
| **Behavioral Task** | **Condition of Performance** | **Frequency or Duration** | **Criteria for Moving to the Next Level of Performance** | **Time Frame** |
| Cover window or mirror with cleaning agent. | -with maximum physical guidance | 1 time per minute | 1 out of 3 times | by: (1 hour) |
| Wipe entire surface with cloth. | -with moderate physical guidance | 3 times per minute | 3 out of 6 times | by: (6 hours) |
| Dry entire surface with cloth or newspaper. | -with minimal physical guidance | 5 times per minute | __ out of __ times | by: (__ hours) |
| Put mirror or window cleaning supplies away following use. | -with ___% physical guidance | 1 time per hour | 4 consecutive trials out of 8 | by: (1 day) |
| | -with tactile cues | 3 times per hour | 12 consecutive trials out of 15 | by: (3 days) |
| **Electrical** | -with a demonstration | 5 times per hour | __ consecutive trials out of __ | by: (__ days) |
| **Light Bulb.** The client will: | -with less than 5 verbal prompts | 6 consecutive times per hour | 20% of the time | by: (1 week) |
| Identify when a light bulb needs to be changed. | -with less than 3 verbal prompts | 2 times per day | 50% of the time | by: (3 weeks) |
| Check to see that light switch is turned off. | -with 1 verbal prompt | 3 times per day | ___% of the time | by: (1 month) |
| Remove fixture and shade if necessary. | -with maximum assistance | 6 times per day | | by: (6 weeks) |
| Check to see that bulb is cool. | -with moderate assistance | 1 time per week | | by: (8 weeks) |
| Turn bulb slowly out of socket. | -with minimum assistance | 3 times per week | | by: (3 months) |
| Throw old bulb in trash. | -with ___% assistance | 8 times per week | | by: (__ months) |
| Obtain a new replacement bulb with appropriate wattage. | -in the therapy setting | 1 time per month | | |
| Place new bulb in socket. | -in the home setting | 3 times per month | | |
| Replace fixture and shade if necessary. | -independently | 6 times per month | | |
| | -safely | | | |

*Table 8-1 (Continued)*

| Household Management | Objective | | | |
|---|---|---|---|---|
| **Behavioral Task** | **Condition of Performance** | **Frequency or Duration** | **Criteria for Moving to the Next Level of Performance** | **Time Frame** |
| **Fuse.** The client will: | | | | |
| Keep flashlight/emergency candles on hand in case of power loss. | -with maximum physical guidance | 1 time per minute | 1 out of 3 times | by: (1 hour) |
| Identify power loss problems to landlord if appropriate. | -with moderate physical guidance | 3 times per minute | 3 out of 6 times | by: (6 hours) |
| Label all circuit breakers in household. | -with minimal physical guidance | 5 times per minute | __ out of __ times | by: (__ hours) |
| Appropriately activate correct switch on circuit breaker following power loss. | -with ___% physical guidance | 1 time per hour | 4 consecutive trials out of 8 | by: (1 day) |
| Label all fuses in the fuse box. | -with tactile cues | 3 times per hour | 12 consecutive trials out of 15 | by: (3 days) |
| Replace fuse in fuse box when loss of power. | -with a demonstration | 5 times per hour | __ consecutive trials out of __ | by: (__ days) |
| Secure an electrician when appropriate. | -with less than 5 verbal prompts | 6 consecutive times per hour | 20% of the time | by: (1 week) |
| **Plumbing.** The client will: | -with less than 3 verbal prompts | 2 times per day | 50% of the time | by: (3 weeks) |
| Put drain cleaner in drains when needed. | -with 1 verbal prompt | 3 times per day | ___% of the time | by: (1 month) |
| Identify problems with plumbing to landlord if appropriate. | -with maximum assistance | 6 times per day | | by: (6 weeks) |
| Replace the washer in a leaky faucet. | -with moderate assistance | 1 time per week | | by: (8 weeks) |
| Use a plunger to unplug a toilet when necessary. | -with minimum assistance | 3 times per week | | by: (3 months) |
| Place only toilet tissue in the bowl for flushing. | -with ___% assistance | 8 times per week | | by: (__ months) |
| | -in the therapy setting | 1 time per month | | |
| | -in the home setting | 3 times per month | | |
| | -independently | 6 times per month | | |
| | -safely | | | |

*Table 8-1 (Continued)*

| Household Management | Objective | | | |
|---|---|---|---|---|
| **Behavioral Task** | **Condition of Performance** | **Frequency or Duration** | **Criteria for Moving to the Next Level of Performance** | **Time Frame** |
| Identify where to turn the water off in the household. | -with maximum physical guidance | 1 time per minute | 1 out of 3 times | by: (1 hour) |
| | -with moderate physical guidance | 3 times per minute | 3 out of 6 times | by: (6 hours) |
| Identify where to turn the water on in the household. | -with minimal physical guidance | 5 times per minute | __ out of __ times | by: (__ hours) |
| Secure a plumber when appropriate. | -with ___% physical guidance | 1 time per hour | 4 consecutive trials out of 8 | by: (1 day) |
| **Interior Maintenance.** The client will: | -with tactile cues | 3 times per hour | 12 consecutive trials out of 15 | by: (3 days) |
| Wipe off finger prints and marks on walls. | -with a demonstration | 5 times per hour | __ consecutive trials out of __ | by: (__ days) |
| Wipe up spills when they occur. | -with less than 5 verbal prompts | 6 consecutive times per hour | 20% of the time | by: (1 week) |
| Identify when screws need to be tightened or replaced in the household. | -with less than 3 verbal prompts | 2 times per day | 50% of the time | by: (3 weeks) |
| | -with 1 verbal prompt | 3 times per day | ___% of the time | by: (1 month) |
| Correctly tighten or replace screws when needed using a screwdriver. | -with maximum assistance | 6 times per day | | by: (6 weeks) |
| Identify when nails need to be hammered or replaced in the household. | -with moderate assistance | 1 time per week | | by: (8 weeks) |
| | -with minimum assistance | 3 times per week | | by: (3 months) |
| Correctly hammer or replace nails using a hammer. | -with ___% assistance | 8 times per week | | by: (__ months) |
| Repair leaky windows and doors during winter months. | -in the therapy setting | 1 time per month | | |
| | -in the home setting | 3 times per month | | |
| Wash window coverings, draperies, and curtains when needed. | -independently | 6 times per month | | |
| Hang pictures or decorative articles on the walls. | | | | |

*Table 8-1 (Continued)*

| Household Management | Objective | | | |
|---|---|---|---|---|
| **Behavioral Task** | **Condition of Performance** | **Frequency or Duration** | **Criteria for Moving to the Next Level of Performance** | **Time Frame** |
| Identify when appliances need to be repaired. | -with maximum physical guidance | 1 time per minute | 1 out of 3 times | by: (1 hour) |
| Replace batteries in household appliances when needed (smoke detectors, radios, flashlights). | -with moderate physical guidance | 3 times per minute | 3 out of 6 times | by: (6 hours) |
| | -with minimal physical guidance | 5 times per minute | __ out of __ times | by: (__ hours) |
| Secure the services of appliance repairperson when appropriate. | -with ___% physical guidance | 1 time per hour | 4 consecutive trials out of 8 | by: (1 day) |
| | -with tactile cues | 3 times per hour | 12 consecutive trials out of 15 | by: (3 days) |
| Identify when painted surfaces need to be repainted or touched up. | -with a demonstration | 5 times per hour | __ consecutive trials out of __ | by: (__ days) |
| Purchase and change furnace filters when needed. | -with less than 5 verbal prompts | 6 consecutive times per hour | 20% of the time | by: (1 week) |
| | -with less than 3 verbal prompts | 2 times per day | 50% of the time | by: (3 weeks) |
| **Exterior Maintenance.** The client will: | -with 1 verbal prompt | 3 times per day | ___% of the time | by: (1 month) |
| Shovel snow off walks when necessary. | -with maximum assistance | 6 times per day | | by: (6 weeks) |
| Clear debris off walks and front stoop. | -with moderate assistance | 1 time per week | | by: (8 weeks) |
| Identify when exterior requires paint or repair. | -with minimum assistance | 3 times per week | | by: (3 months) |
| Secure services from appropriate individuals to paint and repair home. | -with ___% assistance | 8 times per week | | by: (__ months) |
| | -in the therapy setting | 1 time per month | | |
| Put up storm windows or plastic when needed. | -in the home setting | 3 times per month | | |
| **Pet Care.** The client will: | -independently | 6 times per month | | |
| Water and feed pet. | -safely | | | |

*Table 8-1 (Continued)*

| Household Management | Objective | | | |
|---|---|---|---|---|
| **Behavioral Task** | **Condition of Performance** | **Frequency or Duration** | **Criteria for Moving to the Next Level of Performance** | **Time Frame** |
| Change newspaper on floor of bird cage. | | | | |
| Clean fish bowl/tank. | -with maximum physical guidance | 1 time per minute | 1 out of 3 times | by: (1 hour) |
| Let dog outside to toilet. | -with moderate physical guidance | 3 times per minute | 3 out of 6 times | by: (6 hours) |
| Empty litter box. | -with minimal physical guidance | 5 times per minute | __ out of __ times | by: (__ hours) |
| Select a person to care for pet when hospitalized or away. | -with ___% physical guidance | 1 time per hour | 4 consecutive trials out of 8 | by: (1 day) |
| | -with tactile cues | 3 times per hour | 12 consecutive trials out of 15 | by: (3 days) |
| Take pet to vet for maintenance (heartworm pills, shots). | -with a demonstration | 5 times per hour | __ consecutive trials out of __ | by: (__ days) |
| Take pet to vet when ill or injured. | -with less than 5 verbal prompts | 6 consecutive times per hour | 20% of the time | by: (1 week) |
| Purchase food for pet. | -with less than 3 verbal prompts | 2 times per day | 50% of the time | by: (3 weeks) |
| **Plant Care.** The client will: | -with 1 verbal prompt | 3 times per day | ___% of the time | by: (1 month) |
| Identify when plants need to be watered and water them. | -with maximum assistance | 6 times per day | | by: (6 weeks) |
| | -with moderate assistance | 1 time per week | | by: (8 weeks) |
| Place plants in best light in household for growth. | -with minimum assistance | 3 times per week | | by: (3 months) |
| Trim off dead leaves on plants. | -with ___% assistance | 8 times per week | | by: (__ months) |
| Identify when plants need to be fertilized and fertilize them. | -in the therapy setting | 1 time per month | | |
| | -in the home setting | 3 times per month | | |
| Select a person to take care of plants when hospitalized or away. | -independently | 6 times per month | | |

*Table 8-1 (Continued)*

| *Household Management* | | **Objective** | | |
|---|---|---|---|---|
| **Behavioral Task** | **Condition of Performance** | **Frequency or Duration** | **Criteria for Moving to the Next Level of Performance** | **Time Frame** |
| **Childproofing.** The client will: | | | | |
| Place all cleaning supplies in childproof latched cupboards or above the reach of small children. | -with maximum physical guidance | 1 time per minute | 1 out of 3 times | by: (1 hour) |
| | -with moderate physical guidance | 3 times per minute | 3 out of 6 times | by: (6 hours) |
| Place all medicine in childproof latched cupboards or above the reach of small children. | -with minimal physical guidance | 5 times per minute | __ out of __ times | by: (__ hours) |
| | -with ___% physical guidance | 1 time per hour | 4 consecutive trials out of 8 | by: (1 day) |
| Identify plants that are poisonous to adults and children. | -with tactile cues | 3 times per hour | 12 consecutive trials out of 15 | by: (3 days) |
| Cover all electrical outlets with plastic caps. | -with a demonstration | 5 times per hour | __ consecutive trials out of __ | by: (__ days) |
| Store all sharp objects (knives, pencils, pens) out of the reach of small children. | -with less than 5 verbal prompts | 6 consecutive times per hour | 20% of the time | by: (1 week) |
| | -with less than 3 verbal prompts | 2 times per day | 50% of the time | by: (3 weeks) |
| Purchase cleaning supplies and medicine with childproof caps. | -with 1 verbal prompt | 3 times per day | ___% of the time | by: (1 month) |
| | -with maximum assistance | 6 times per day | | by: (6 weeks) |
| Store all flammable liquids out of the reach of small children (gasoline, kerosene, paint supplies). | -with moderate assistance | 1 time per week | | by: (8 weeks) |
| Store all cleaning supplies and flammable liquids in containers that did not store edible objects or drinks (beverage bottles, milk cartons). | -with minimum assistance | 3 times per week | | by: (3 months) |
| | -with ___% assistance | 8 times per week | | by: (__ months) |
| Store matches and lighters out of the reach of children. | -in the therapy setting | 1 time per month | | |
| | -in the home setting | 3 times per month | | |
| Keep smoking materials (ashtrays, lighters, cigarettes) away from children. | -independently | 6 times per month | | |
| Keep a Poison Control hotline number near the telephone. | -safely | | | |

© SLACK Inc.

## Therapeutic Suggestions

1. Have clients look in newspapers for rental units that meet individual requirements of cost, location, and space.

2. Practice filling out applications for apartments.

3. Discuss the pros and cons of having roommates. What type of personality would the client want to live with?

4. Discuss the pros and cons of living in Adult Foster Care.

5. Discuss the qualifications and application process for subsidized housing.

6. Discuss the type of rental unit that can be obtained on limited income.

7. Have client make an appointment to have a rental unit shown.

8. Discuss legal ways of evicting people and what can be done to prevent this from happening.

9. Discuss the costs of apartment living versus buying your own home. Which is more expensive?

10. Provide client with a daily checklist to maintain personal space (clothing picked up, magazines put away).

11. Discuss how to organize cupboards and closets for ease in finding objects and clothing.

12. Make a list and identify cost of all cleaning supplies needed to maintain a household.

13. Provide a daily log or calendar to record what needs to be cleaned which also provides a visual means of identifying what has already been cleaned.

14. Organize a "fix it" group where each client has to identify and fix something that needs repair.

15. Invite an electrician to the group to talk about how to replace a fuse, operate a circuit breaker, and change a furnace filter. Also discuss safe and unsafe wiring.

16. Rent videos available on interior and exterior maintenance (Better Homes and Gardens) and discuss the importance of these activities.

17. Discuss the care and maintenance of pets including cost, supplies, equipment needed, and health requirements.

18. Organize a gardening group where each client is responsible for the survival of a plant, flower, or vegetable.

19. Discuss poison prevention including poisonous plants. Obtain information from a poison control center.

20. Discuss ways of baby proofing a household and identify childproof cupboard latches and electrical caps that are commercially available.

21. Discuss inexpensive ways of making a home attractive through decorating (curtains, pictures, lighting, color, texture).

22. Discuss inexpensive ways of furnishing an apartment or home (garage sales, thrift shops, going out-of-business sales).

# Chapter 9

# Leisure Planning

The purpose of this chapter is to identify various behavioral components necessary for leisure planning. It is important for individuals to cope with and determine what to do during unoccupied time, to expand opportunities for social interaction and community involvement.

When looking at leisure planning, one must first explore all possible activities available in the home and community environment. Then preferences, interests, and values assist an individual in making choices. Once activities are chosen, issues of affordability and access must be resolved. Finally, the activity has to be initiated, attended to, and ended at an appropriate time. Leisure planning allows opportunities for social interactions and relationships, enhancing quality of life.

*Table 9-1*

| Leisure Planning | | | Objective | |
|---|---|---|---|---|
| **Behavioral Task** | **Condition of Performance** | **Frequency or Duration** | **Criteria for Moving to the Next Level of Performance** | **Time Frame** |
| **Play or Leisure Exploration.** The client will: | | | | |
| Identify recreational activities one can do in the community. | -with maximum physical guidance | 1 time per minute | 1 out of 3 times | by: (1 hour) |
| | -with moderate physical guidance | 3 times per minute | 3 out of 6 times | by: (6 hours) |
| Identify recreational activities that require participation (dancing). | -with minimal physical guidance | 5 times per minute | __ out of __ times | by: (__ hours) |
| Identify recreational activities that are non-participatory. | -with ___% physical guidance | 1 time per hour | 4 consecutive trials out of 8 | by: (1 day) |
| | -with tactile cues | 3 times per hour | 12 consecutive trials out of 15 | by: (3 days) |
| Identify recreational activities that cost money. | -with a demonstration | 5 times per hour | __ consecutive trials out of __ | by: (__ days) |
| Identify recreational activities that are free. | -with less than 5 verbal prompts | 6 consecutive times per hour | 20% of the time | by: (1 week) |
| Identify recreational activities that require equipment (skiing, tennis, golf). | -with less than 3 verbal prompts | 2 times per day | 50% of the time | by: (3 weeks) |
| Identify recreational activities that one can do with others. | -with 1 verbal prompt | 3 times per day | ___% of the time | by: (1 month) |
| | -with maximum assistance | 6 times per day | | by: (6 weeks) |
| Identify recreational activities that one can do alone. | -with moderate assistance | 1 time per week | | by: (8 weeks) |
| | -with minimum assistance | 3 times per week | | by: (3 months) |
| Identify clubs or organized social activities for possible participation. | -with ___% assistance | 8 times per week | | by: (__ months) |
| Identify preferred recreational activities from a list. | -in the therapy setting | 1 time per month | | |
| | -in the home setting | 3 times per month | | |
| Identify preferred hobbies. | -in a community setting | 6 times per month | | |
| Identify preferred spectator activities. | -independently | | | |

© SLACK Inc.

*Table 9-1 (Continued)*

| Leisure Planning | Objective | | | |
|---|---|---|---|---|
| **Behavioral Task** | **Condition of Performance** | **Frequency or Duration** | **Criteria for Moving to the Next Level of Performance** | **Time Frame** |
| Identify preferred table games. | -with maximum physical guidance | 1 time per minute | 1 out of 3 times | by: (1 hour) |
| Identify preferred sport participation activities. | -with moderate physical guidance | 3 times per minute | 3 out of 6 times | by: (6 hours) |
| Identify preferred arts and crafts activities. | -with minimal physical guidance | 5 times per minute | __ out of __ times | by: (__ hours) |
| Identify preferred music. | -with ___% physical guidance | 1 time per hour | 4 consecutive trials out of 8 | by: (1 day) |
| Identify preferred television programs. | -with tactile cues | 3 times per hour | 12 consecutive trials out of 15 | by: (3 days) |
| Seek out leisure time activities. | -with a demonstration | 5 times per hour | __ consecutive trials out of __ | by: (__ days) |
| **Play or Leisure Performance.** | -with less than 5 verbal prompts | 6 consecutive times per hour | 20% of the time | by: (1 week) |
| The client will: | -with less than 3 verbal prompts | 2 times per day | 50% of the time | by: (3 weeks) |
| | -with 1 verbal prompt | 3 times per day | ___% of the time | by: (1 month) |
| Discriminate leisure time from work time. | -with maximum assistance | 6 times per day | | by: (6 weeks) |
| Schedule leisure time. | -with moderate assistance | 1 time per week | | by: (8 weeks) |
| Choose from presented activities for leisure time. | -with minimum assistance | 3 times per week | | by: (3 months) |
| Initiate leisure time activity. | -with ___% assistance | 8 times per week | | by: (__ months) |
| Attend to chosen leisure time activity. | -in the therapy setting | 1 time per month | | |
| End leisure activity when time is up. | -in the home setting | 3 times per month | | |
| Clean-up area following leisure time activity. | -independently | 6 times per month | | |
| Put away supplies, equipment, and materials following leisure time activity. | | | | |
| Respect the rights and property of others engaged in leisure time activity. | | | | |

*Table 9-1 (Continued)*

| Leisure Planning | | Objective | | |
|---|---|---|---|---|
| **Behavioral Task** | **Condition of Performance** | **Frequency or Duration** | **Criteria for Moving to the Next Level of Performance** | **Time Frame** |
| Exhibit good sportsmanship during leisure time activity. | -with maximum physical guidance | 1 time per minute | 1 out of 3 times | by: (1 hour) |
| | -with moderate physical guidance | 3 times per minute | 3 out of 6 times | by: (6 hours) |
| Help plan a recreational activity with a group. | -with minimal physical guidance | 5 times per minute | __ out of __ times | by: (__ hours) |
| Take part in a recreational activity planned by a group. | -with ___% physical guidance | 1 time per hour | 4 consecutive trials out of 8 | by: (1 day) |
| | -with tactile cues | 3 times per hour | 12 consecutive trials out of 15 | by: (3 days) |
| Plan free recreational activities for oneself. | -with a demonstration | 5 times per hour | __ consecutive trials out of __ | by: (__ days) |
| Choose and pay for one participatory activity. | -with less than 5 verbal prompts | 6 consecutive times per hour | 20% of the time | by: (1 week) |
| Choose and pay for one non-participatory activity. | -with less than 3 verbal prompts | 2 times per day | 50% of the time | by: (3 weeks) |
| | -with 1 verbal prompt | 3 times per day | ___% of the time | by: (1 month) |
| Make plans with friends to attend activities outside the home. | -with maximum assistance | 6 times per day | | by: (6 weeks) |
| Organize a recreational activity at own residence (cards, games). | -with moderate assistance | 1 time per week | | by: (8 weeks) |
| | -with minimum assistance | 3 times per week | | by: (3 months) |
| Plan for and entertain others at home. | -with ___% assistance | 8 times per week | | by: (__ months) |
| Join and participate in organized social activities (clubs or teams). | -in the therapy setting | 1 time per month | | |
| Plan and budget for two paid recreational activities with one friend, and execute them appropriately. | -in the home setting | 3 times per month | | |
| | -in a community setting | 6 times per month | | |
| Plan, budget, and execute a weekend of recreation from Friday evening through Sunday. | -independently | | | |

*Table 9-1 (Continued)*

| Leisure Planning | Objective | | | |
|---|---|---|---|---|
| **Behavioral Task** | **Condition of Performance** | **Frequency or Duration** | **Criteria for Moving to the Next Level of Performance** | **Time Frame** |
| **Spectator Activities.** The client will: | | | | |
| Plan in advance to attend a spectator activity (theatre, baseball game). | -with maximum physical guidance | 1 time per minute | 1 out of 3 times | by: (1 hour) |
| | -with moderate physical guidance | 3 times per minute | 3 out of 6 times | by: (6 hours) |
| Ask a friend to attend the spectator activity. | -with minimal physical guidance | 5 times per minute | __ out of __ times | by: (__ hours) |
| Budget money in advance for spectator activity (theatre, baseball game). | -with ___% physical guidance | 1 time per hour | 4 consecutive trials out of 8 | by: (1 day) |
| Purchase tickets in advance for a spectator activity if appropriate. | -with tactile cues | 3 times per hour | 12 consecutive trials out of 15 | by: (3 days) |
| | -with a demonstration | 5 times per hour | __ consecutive trials out of __ | by: (__ days) |
| Arrive at a spectator activity on time. | -with less than 5 verbal prompts | 6 consecutive times per hour | 20% of the time | by: (1 week) |
| Attend to the spectator activity. | -with less than 3 verbal prompts | 2 times per day | 50% of the time | by: (3 weeks) |
| Remain at a spectator activity for the duration. | -with 1 verbal prompt | 3 times per day | ___% of the time | by: (1 month) |
| Engage in appropriate audience behavior. | -with maximum assistance | 6 times per day | | by: (6 weeks) |
| **Sport Participation Activities.** The client will: | -with moderate assistance | 1 time per week | | by: (8 weeks) |
| | -with minimum assistance | 3 times per week | | by: (3 months) |
| Dress appropriately to participate in the sport. | -with ___% assistance | 8 times per week | | by: (__ months) |
| Secure equipment needed to participate in the sport. | -in the therapy setting | 1 time per month | | |
| Budget in advance to participate in the sport. | -in the home setting | 3 times per month | | |
| Identify the rules of the sport. | -in a community setting | 6 times per month | | |
| Abide by the rules of the sport during play. | -independently | | | |

*Table 9-1 (Continued)*

| Leisure Planning | Objective | | | |
|---|---|---|---|---|
| **Behavioral Task** | **Condition of Performance** | **Frequency or Duration** | **Criteria for Moving to the Next Level of Performance** | **Time Frame** |
| Secure other players to participate in the sport. | -with maximum physical guidance | 1 time per minute | 1 out of 3 times | by: (1 hour) |
| Organize a sport event. | -with moderate physical guidance | 3 times per minute | 3 out of 6 times | by: (6 hours) |
| **Games.** The client will: | -with minimal physical guidance | 5 times per minute | __ out of __ times | by: (__ hours) |
| Obtain equipment or pieces to set up a game. | -with ___% physical guidance | 1 time per hour | 4 consecutive trials out of 8 | by: (1 day) |
| | -with tactile cues | 3 times per hour | 12 consecutive trials out of 15 | by: (3 days) |
| Secure additional players to play a game. | -with a demonstration | 5 times per hour | __ consecutive trials out of __ | by: (__ days) |
| Identify how to play a game. | -with less than 5 verbal prompts | 6 consecutive times per hour | 20% of the time | by: (1 week) |
| Identify the rules of the game. | -with less than 3 verbal prompts | 2 times per day | 50% of the time | by: (3 weeks) |
| Proceed through steps of game. | -with 1 verbal prompt | 3 times per day | ___% of the time | by: (1 month) |
| Assist others in playing the game if needed. | -with maximum assistance | 6 times per day | | by: (6 weeks) |
| Wait his turn during the game. | -with moderate assistance | 1 time per week | | by: (8 weeks) |
| **Hobbies.** The client will: | -with minimum assistance | 3 times per week | | by: (3 months) |
| Identify potential choices for hobbies. | -with ___% assistance | 8 times per week | | by: (__ months) |
| Choose a leisure activity to pursue as a hobby. | -in the therapy setting | 1 time per month | | |
| Obtain information about chosen hobby. | -in the home setting | 3 times per month | | |
| Plan time to work on a hobby. | -in a community setting | 6 times per month | | |
| Work on a hobby. | -independently | | | |
| Complete a hobby in a timely way. | | | | |

*Table 9-1 (Continued)*

| *Leisure Planning* | Objective | | | |
|---|---|---|---|---|
| **Behavioral Task** | **Condition of Performance** | **Frequency or Duration** | **Criteria for Moving to the Next Level of Performance** | **Time Frame** |
| Initiate an additional hobby when one is completed. | -with maximum physical guidance | 1 time per minute | 1 out of 3 times | by: (1 hour) |
| | -with moderate physical guidance | 3 times per minute | 3 out of 6 times | by: (6 hours) |
| Budget money to purchase items for a hobby. | -with minimal physical guidance | 5 times per minute | __ out of __ times | by: (__ hours) |
| **Arts and Crafts.** The client will: | -with ___% physical guidance | 1 time per hour | 4 consecutive trials out of 8 | by: (1 day) |
| Obtain materials, supplies, and instruction for completing an art/craft activity. | -with tactile cues | 3 times per hour | 12 consecutive trials out of 15 | by: (3 days) |
| Initiate an art/craft activity. | -with a demonstration | 5 times per hour | __ consecutive trials out of __ | by: (__ days) |
| Follow directions for an art/craft activity. | -with less than 5 verbal prompts | 6 consecutive times per hour | 20% of the time | by: (1 week) |
| Determine when an art/craft activity is completed. | -with less than 3 verbal prompts | 2 times per day | 50% of the time | by: (3 weeks) |
| | -with 1 verbal prompt | 3 times per day | ___% of the time | by: (1 month) |
| Clean up supplies and materials following an art/craft activity. | -with maximum assistance | 6 times per day | | by: (6 weeks) |
| Organize an art/craft activity with another person. | -with moderate assistance | 1 time per week | | by: (8 weeks) |
| | -with minimum assistance | 3 times per week | | by: (3 months) |
| **Music.** The client will: | -with ___% assistance | 8 times per week | | by: (__ months) |
| Play music on an instrument. | -in the therapy setting | 1 time per month | | |
| Take music lessons. | -in the home setting | 3 times per month | | |
| Listen to music. | -in a community setting | 6 times per month | | |
| Show consideration for others when adjusting volume on radio, record player, tape. | -independently | | | |

*Table 9-1 (Continued)*

| Leisure Planning | Objective | | | |
|---|---|---|---|---|
| **Behavioral Task** | **Condition of Performance** | **Frequency or Duration** | **Criteria for Moving to the Next Level of Performance** | **Time Frame** |
| **Television.**  The client will: | | | | |
| Select preferred programs on television. | -with maximum physical guidance | 1 time per minute | 1 out of 3 times | by: (1 hour) |
| Turn television control to preferred channel. | -with moderate physical guidance | 3 times per minute | 3 out of 6 times | by: (6 hours) |
| Show consideration for others' viewing preferences. | -with minimal physical guidance | 5 times per minute | __ out of __ times | by: (__ hours) |
| | -with ___% physical guidance | 1 time per hour | 4 consecutive trials out of 8 | by: (1 day) |
| Show consideration for others when adjusting volume on the television. | -with tactile cues | 3 times per hour | 12 consecutive trials out of 15 | by: (3 days) |
| | -with a demonstration | 5 times per hour | __ consecutive trials out of __ | by: (__ days) |
| | -with less than 5 verbal prompts | 6 consecutive times per hour | 20% of the time | by: (1 week) |
| | -with less than 3 verbal prompts | 2 times per day | 50% of the time | by: (3 weeks) |
| | -with 1 verbal prompt | 3 times per day | ___% of the time | by: (1 month) |
| | -with maximum assistance | 6 times per day | | by: (6 weeks) |
| | -with moderate assistance | 1 time per week | | by: (8 weeks) |
| | -with minimum assistance | 3 times per week | | by: (3 months) |
| | -with ___% assistance | 8 times per week | | by: (__ months) |
| | -in the therapy setting | 1 time per month | | |
| | -in the home setting | 3 times per month | | |
| | -independently | 6 times per month | | |

## Therapeutic Suggestions

1. Have the group research leisure opportunities in the community that are free versus paid. Look in newspaper entertainment sections and get materials from the local chamber of commerce or tourism bureau.

2. Look at access to community leisure activities. Are they on the bus route; within walking distance?

3. Discuss cost of leisure activities.

4. Have the group look into clubs, organizations, or support groups and discuss which ones they might be interested in joining.

5. Have each group member invite a friend to attend a community meeting of a club, organization, or support group.

6. Conduct a music appreciation group where a variety of different types of music is played. Have group members discuss preference regarding composer, band, instrumentals, etc.

7. Discuss proper audience etiquette for the theatre, spectator sports, movies, etc.

8. Discuss proper dress for the theatre, spectator sports, etc.

9. Conduct a soap opera viewing group and discuss personal problems of the characters and how they cope with them. Have clients identify how they would react in similar situations.

10. Conduct a public broadcasting viewing group on various topics such as the arts, environment, nature, and history followed by discussion.

11. Plan group outings to community activities that are free.

12. Plan group outings to community activities that charge fees.

13. Present information and materials on a variety of hobbies. Have group participants indicate which activities appear interesting. Encourage each group participant to start one hobby.

# Chapter 10

# Social Interaction Skills

The purpose of this chapter is to provide a variety of objectives and techniques developed to improve independent living skills in the area of socialization. This chapter covers the area of self-identification and social conduct which encompasses manners, conversation, assertiveness, and developing friendships/relationships. Individuals who receive mental health services often can benefit from social skills training. Social skills directly affect all areas of independent living. Communicating individual wants and needs is very important when receiving health services. The services that are received often depend on the manner in which the request was made.

Social skills frequently are environment specific in that behaviors displayed at home may not be accepted in a school, work, or church setting. To decide what is and what is not acceptable can be a judgment call by the individual. Persons receiving health services may demonstrate difficulty in judging what is acceptable behavior. To assist individuals in developing skills in social situations, training is very important and may require repeated sessions before behavior change occurs. This area may be provided to individuals who demonstrate the inability to interact positively with others. Providing social skills training will increase the ability for others to live independently and improve the quality of life.

*Table 10-1*

| Social Interaction Skills | Objective | | | |
|---|---|---|---|---|
| **Behavioral Task** | **Condition of Performance** | **Frequency or Duration** | **Criteria for Moving to the Next Level of Performance** | **Time Frame** |
| **Self Identification.** The client will: | | | | |
| Recognize personal and non-personal information. | -with maximum physical guidance | 1 time per minute | 1 out of 3 times | by: (1 hour) |
| | -with moderate physical guidance | 3 times per minute | 3 out of 6 times | by: (6 hours) |
| Provide personal information (name, birth date, address) verbally and written when asked. | -with minimal physical guidance | 5 times per minute | __ out of __ times | by: (__ hours) |
| | -with ___% physical guidance | 1 time per hour | 4 consecutive trials out of 8 | by: (1 day) |
| Verbalize and improve personal strengths and weaknesses. | -with tactile cues | 3 times per hour | 12 consecutive trials out of 15 | by: (3 days) |
| Verbalize similarities and differences in self and others. | -with a demonstration | 5 times per hour | __ consecutive trials out of __ | by: (__ days) |
| | -with less than 5 verbal prompts | 6 consecutive times per hour | 20% of the time | by: (1 week) |
| Develop realistic personal and professional goals. | -with less than 3 verbal prompts | 2 times per day | 50% of the time | by: (3 weeks) |
| Develop a plan to achieve personal and professional goals. | -with 1 verbal prompt | 3 times per day | ___% of the time | by: (1 month) |
| | -with maximum assistance | 6 times per day | | by: (6 weeks) |
| Follow a plan developed to achieve goals. | -with moderate assistance | 1 time per week | | by: (8 weeks) |
| Verbalize positive and negative outcomes of the plan. | -with minimum assistance | 3 times per week | | by: (3 months) |
| Take pride in personal accomplishments. | -with ___% assistance | 8 times per week | | by: (__ months) |
| Continue to try after experiencing failure. | -in the therapy setting | 1 time per month | | |
| Revise the plan to achieve goals when necessary. | -in the home setting | 3 times per month | | |
| Work and interact with others cooperatively. | -independently | 6 times per month | | |

*Table 10-1 (Continued)*

| Social Interaction Skills | **Objective** | | | |
|---|---|---|---|---|

| Behavioral Task | Condition of Performance | Frequency or Duration | Criteria for Moving to the Next Level of Performance | Time Frame |
|---|---|---|---|---|
| **Social Conduct.** The client will: | | | | |
| Identify courteous and non-courteous behavior. | -with maximum physical guidance | 1 time per minute | 1 out of 3 times | by: (1 hour) |
| | -with moderate physical guidance | 3 times per minute | 3 out of 6 times | by: (6 hours) |
| Greet others by name, shaking hands when necessary. | -with minimal physical guidance | 5 times per minute | __ out of __ times | by: (__ hours) |
| Verbalize "please" when making requests and "thank you" when receiving items or assistance. | -with ___% physical guidance | 1 time per hour | 4 consecutive trials out of 8 | by: (1 day) |
| | -with tactile cues | 3 times per hour | 12 consecutive trials out of 15 | by: (3 days) |
| Chew gum politely. | -with a demonstration | 5 times per hour | __ consecutive trials out of __ | by: (__ days) |
| Cover mouth when yawning or coughing. | -with less than 5 verbal prompts | 6 consecutive times per hour | 20% of the time | by: (1 week) |
| Assist others to improve courteous behavior. | -with less than 3 verbal prompts | 2 times per day | 50% of the time | by: (3 weeks) |
| Improve courteous behaviors in self. | -with 1 verbal prompt | 3 times per day | ___% of the time | by: (1 month) |
| Perform in a socially acceptable manner in specific environments (church, school, work, and as a guest). | -with maximum assistance | 6 times per day | | by: (6 weeks) |
| | -with moderate assistance | 1 time per week | | by: (8 weeks) |
| Identify and practice rules of cooperating with others. | -with minimum assistance | 3 times per week | | by: (3 months) |
| **Table Manners.** The client will: | -with ___% assistance | 8 times per week | | by: (__ months) |
| Demonstrate correct posture when sitting. | -in the therapy setting | 1 time per month | | |
| Place napkin on lap and use when necessary. | -in the home setting | 3 times per month | | |
| Use eating utensils when necessary. | -in a restaurant setting | 6 times per month | | |
| Use eating utensils accurately. | -in a public setting | | | |
| | -independently | | | |

© SLACK Inc.

81

*Table 10-1 (Continued)*

| Social Interaction Skills | Objective | | | |
|---|---|---|---|---|
| **Behavioral Task** | **Condition of Performance** | **Frequency or Duration** | **Criteria for Moving to the Next Level of Performance** | **Time Frame** |
| Eat finger food correctly. | -with maximum physical guidance | 1 time per minute | 1 out of 3 times | by: (1 hour) |
| Eat one food item with one hand. | -with moderate physical guidance | 3 times per minute | 3 out of 6 times | by: (6 hours) |
| Identify between proper and improper table manners. | -with minimal physical guidance | 5 times per minute | __ out of __ times | by: (__ hours) |
| | -with ___% physical guidance | 1 time per hour | 4 consecutive trials out of 8 | by: (1 day) |
| Take proper-sized portions of food and beverages. | -with tactile cues | 3 times per hour | 12 consecutive trials out of 15 | by: (3 days) |
| Take proper-sized bites of food. | -with a demonstration | 5 times per hour | __ consecutive trials out of __ | by: (__ days) |
| Consume proper amount of beverages. | -with less than 5 verbal prompts | 6 consecutive times per hour | 20% of the time | by: (1 week) |
| Pass food or beverages when asked. | -with less than 3 verbal prompts | 2 times per day | 50% of the time | by: (3 weeks) |
| Ask permission to have second helpings. | -with 1 verbal prompt | 3 times per day | ___% of the time | by: (1 month) |
| Verbalize "please" and "thank you" when requesting or receiving items or assistance. | -with maximum assistance | 6 times per day | | by: (6 weeks) |
| | -with moderate assistance | 1 time per week | | by: (8 weeks) |
| Chew food with mouth closed. | -with minimum assistance | 3 times per week | | by: (3 months) |
| Talk without food in mouth. | -with ___% assistance | 8 times per week | | by: (__ months) |
| Cover mouth when coughing, burping, etc. | -in the therapy setting | 1 time per month | | |
| Discard food items that fall on floor. | -in the home setting | 3 times per month | | |
| Eat meal in reasonable amount of time. | -in a restaurant setting | 6 times per month | | |
| Engage in dinner conversation. | -independently | | | |
| Stay seated at table until all dinner guests are finished eating. | | | | |

© SLACK Inc.

*Table 10-1 (Continued)*

| Social Interaction Skills | Objective | | | |
|---|---|---|---|---|
| **Behavioral Task** | **Condition of Performance** | **Frequency or Duration** | **Criteria for Moving to the Next Level of Performance** | **Time Frame** |
| Smoke only if all dinner guests give permission. | -with maximum physical guidance | 1 time per minute | 1 out of 3 times | by: (1 hour) |
| Excuse self from table. | -with moderate physical guidance | 3 times per minute | 3 out of 6 times | by: (6 hours) |
| Thank individual who prepared the meal. | -with minimal physical guidance | 5 times per minute | __ out of __ times | by: (__ hours) |
| Offer assistance in cleaning up after the meal. | -with ___% physical guidance | 1 time per hour | 4 consecutive trials out of 8 | by: (1 day) |
| Use table manners when dining out. | -with tactile cues | 3 times per hour | 12 consecutive trials out of 15 | by: (3 days) |
| | -with a demonstration | 5 times per hour | __ consecutive trials out of __ | by: (__ days) |
| **Conversation.** The client will: | -with less than 5 verbal prompts | 6 consecutive times per hour | 20% of the time | by: (1 week) |
| Identify self and others by name. | -with less than 3 verbal prompts | 2 times per day | 50% of the time | by: (3 weeks) |
| Maintain eye contact with others. | -with 1 verbal prompt | 3 times per day | ___% of the time | by: (1 month) |
| Smile at others when greeting them. | -with maximum assistance | 6 times per day | | by: (6 weeks) |
| Display verbal and nonverbal gestures when greeting others and saying "goodbye." | -with moderate assistance | 1 time per week | | by: (8 weeks) |
| Converse with others at arm's-length distance. | -with minimum assistance | 3 times per week | | by: (3 months) |
| Pronounce words clearly. | -with ___% assistance | 8 times per week | | by: (__ months) |
| Speak in whole sentences. | -in the therapy setting | 1 time per month | | |
| Speak in a sequence that is understandable to others. | -in the home setting | 3 times per month | | |
| Speak when others are visually present. | -in a restaurant setting | 6 times per month | | |
| Use facial expressions to communicate during conversation. | -independently | | | |

© SLACK Inc.

*Table 10-1 (Continued)*

| Social Interaction Skills | | | | Objective |
|---|---|---|---|---|
| **Behavioral Task** | **Condition of Performance** | **Frequency or Duration** | **Criteria for Moving to the Next Level of Performance** | **Time Frame** |
| Speak at a speed where others are able to understand the content of the conversation. | -with maximum physical guidance | 1 time per minute | 1 out of 3 times | by: (1 hour) |
| | -with moderate physical guidance | 3 times per minute | 3 out of 6 times | by: (6 hours) |
| Speak in a voice volume that is conducive to the environment. | -with minimal physical guidance | 5 times per minute | __ out of __ times | by: (__ hours) |
| Speak faster or slower as needed. | -with ___% physical guidance | 1 time per hour | 4 consecutive trials out of 8 | by: (1 day) |
| Listen to others without interrupting. | -with tactile cues | 3 times per hour | 12 consecutive trials out of 15 | by: (3 days) |
| Practice active listening with one person and in a group. | -with a demonstration | 5 times per hour | __ consecutive trials out of __ | by: (__ days) |
| Respond to humor and jokes with a smile or laugh when necessary. | -with less than 5 verbal prompts | 6 consecutive times per hour | 20% of the time | by: (1 week) |
| | -with less than 3 verbal prompts | 2 times per day | 50% of the time | by: (3 weeks) |
| Ask and answer questions related to the topic at hand. | -with 1 verbal prompt | 3 times per day | ___% of the time | by: (1 month) |
| | -with maximum assistance | 6 times per day | | by: (6 weeks) |
| Engage in relevant conversation with others. | -with moderate assistance | 1 time per week | | by: (8 weeks) |
| Initiate and maintain conversation. | -with minimum assistance | 3 times per week | | by: (3 months) |
| End conversations when necessary. | -with ___% assistance | 8 times per week | | by: (__ months) |
| Learn American Sign Language as needed. | -in the therapy setting | 1 time per month | | |
| Use American Sign Language as needed. | -in the home setting | 3 times per month | | |
| Teach others to use American Sign Language. | -in a public setting | 6 times per month | | |
| Verbalize how communication patterns effect others. | -independently | | | |

© SLACK Inc.

*Table 10-1 (Continued)*

| Social Interaction Skills | Objective | | | |
|---|---|---|---|---|
| **Behavioral Task** | **Condition of Performance** | **Frequency or Duration** | **Criteria for Moving to the Next Level of Performance** | **Time Frame** |
| Verbalize how own communication patterns effect others. | -with maximum physical guidance | 1 time per minute | 1 out of 3 times | by: (1 hour) |
| | -with moderate physical guidance | 3 times per minute | 3 out of 6 times | by: (6 hours) |
| **Telephone Skills.** The client will: | -with minimal physical guidance | 5 times per minute | __ out of __ times | by: (__ hours) |
| Identify parts of telephone and use correctly. | -with ___% physical guidance | 1 time per hour | 4 consecutive trials out of 8 | by: (1 day) |
| Identify and demonstrate how to use pay phone. | -with tactile cues | 3 times per hour | 12 consecutive trials out of 15 | by: (3 days) |
| Pick up receiver when phone rings and greet caller. | -with a demonstration | 5 times per hour | __ consecutive trials out of __ | by: (__ days) |
| Take phone messages for others. | -with less than 5 verbal prompts | 6 consecutive times per hour | 20% of the time | by: (1 week) |
| Maintain conversation on phone. | -with less than 3 verbal prompts | 2 times per day | 50% of the time | by: (3 weeks) |
| End conversation on phone. | -with 1 verbal prompt | 3 times per day | ___% of the time | by: (1 month) |
| Call others on phone and initiate conversation. | -with maximum assistance | 6 times per day | | by: (6 weeks) |
| | -with moderate assistance | 1 time per week | | by: (8 weeks) |
| Verbalize services operator provides. | -with minimum assistance | 3 times per week | | by: (3 months) |
| Verbalize and demonstrate how to use phone book. | -with ___% assistance | 8 times per week | | by: (__ months) |
| Verbalize and demonstrate how to call information for local and out-of-state phone numbers. | -in the therapy setting | 1 time per month | | |
| | -in the home setting | 3 times per month | | |
| | -in a community setting | 6 times per month | | |
| Identify and verbalize difference between local and long distance calling. | -independently | | | |

*Table 10-1 (Continued)*

| Social Interaction Skills | Objective | | | |
|---|---|---|---|---|

| **Behavioral Task** | **Condition of Performance** | **Frequency or Duration** | **Criteria for Moving to the Next Level of Performance** | **Time Frame** |
|---|---|---|---|---|
| **Assertiveness.** The client will: | | | | |
| Verbalize definitions and differences between non-assertive/passive, assertive, passive, and aggressive behavior. | -with maximum physical guidance | 1 time per minute | 1 out of 3 times | by: (1 hour) |
| | -with moderate physical guidance | 3 times per minute | 3 out of 6 times | by: (6 hours) |
| Verbalize how individual rights relate to assertive behavior. | -with minimal physical guidance | 5 times per minute | __ out of __ times | by: (__ hours) |
| | -with ___% physical guidance | 1 time per hour | 4 consecutive trials out of 8 | by: (1 day) |
| Identify own personal rights and verbalize how these rights are equal to others. | -with tactile cues | 3 times per hour | 12 consecutive trials out of 15 | by: (3 days) |
| Voice personal rights in an assertive manner. | -with a demonstration | 5 times per hour | __ consecutive trials out of __ | by: (__ days) |
| Verbalize importance of assertive philosophy. | -with less than 5 verbal prompts | 6 consecutive times per hour | 20% of the time | by: (1 week) |
| Report reasons why people are non-assertive/passive (fear of acceptance). | -with less than 3 verbal prompts | 2 times per day | 50% of the time | by: (3 weeks) |
| | -with 1 verbal prompt | 3 times per day | ___% of the time | by: (1 month) |
| Verbalize consequences of non-assertive/ passive, assertive, and aggressive behaviors. | -with maximum assistance | 6 times per day | | by: (6 weeks) |
| Report non-verbal cues of non-assertive/ passive, assertive and aggressive communication. | -with moderate assistance | 1 time per week | | by: (8 weeks) |
| | -with minimum assistance | 3 times per week | | by: (3 months) |
| Practice and perform important qualities of assertive behavior (eye contact, facial expression, body posture, vocal tone, timing of response, and content of words). | -with ___% assistance | 8 times per week | | by: (__ months) |
| | -in the therapy setting | 1 time per month | | |
| | -in the home setting | 3 times per month | | |
| State definition of active listening and practice this skill. | -independently | 6 times per month | | |

*Table 10-1 (Continued)*

| Social Interaction Skills | **Objective** | | | |
|---|---|---|---|---|

| Behavioral Task | Condition of Performance | Frequency or Duration | Criteria for Moving to the Next Level of Performance | Time Frame |
|---|---|---|---|---|
| Recognize and report verbal behaviors that interfere with active listening (ordering, directions, criticizing, preaching, arguing, blaming, and threatening). | -with maximum physical guidance | 1 time per minute | 1 out of 3 times | by: (1 hour) |
| | -with moderate physical guidance | 3 times per minute | 3 out of 6 times | by: (6 hours) |
| | -with minimal physical guidance | 5 times per minute | __ out of __ times | by: (__ hours) |
| Practice assertion skills by verbalizing feelings employing "I" messages. | -with ___% physical guidance | 1 time per hour | 4 consecutive trials out of 8 | by: (1 day) |
| Report how the use of "you" statements contradict assertive philosophy. | -with tactile cues | 3 times per hour | 12 consecutive trials out of 15 | by: (3 days) |
| | -with a demonstration | 5 times per hour | __ consecutive trials out of __ | by: (__ days) |
| Practice assertive behavior when making and denying requests. | -with less than 5 verbal prompts | 6 consecutive times per hour | 20% of the time | by: (1 week) |
| Demonstrate and practice responding assertively to others who demand or nag. | -with less than 3 verbal prompts | 2 times per day | 50% of the time | by: (3 weeks) |
| Demonstrate and practice confrontation skills in an assertive manner. | -with 1 verbal prompt | 3 times per day | ___% of the time | by: (1 month) |
| | -with maximum assistance | 6 times per day | | by: (6 weeks) |
| Verbalize importance of accepting responsibility for own behaviors. | -with moderate assistance | 1 time per week | | by: (8 weeks) |
| | -with minimum assistance | 3 times per week | | by: (3 months) |
| Verbalize importance of not accepting responsibility for others' behavior. | -with ___% assistance | 8 times per week | | by: (__ months) |
| Avoid apologizing for behavior not caused by self. | -in the therapy setting | 1 time per month | | |
| | -in the home setting | 3 times per month | | |
| Verbalize and practice how to manage authoritarian behavior with assertive skills. | -independently | 6 times per month | | |
| Verbalize and practice how to request time and information from busy professionals. | | | | |

*Table 10-1 (Continued)*

| Social Interaction Skills | | Objective | | |
|---|---|---|---|---|
| **Behavioral Task** | **Condition of Performance** | **Frequency or Duration** | **Criteria for Moving to the Next Level of Performance** | **Time Frame** |
| Verbalize and practice how to request a medication change from a physician or psychiatrist. | -with maximum physical guidance | 1 time per minute | 1 out of 3 times | by: (1 hour) |
| | -with moderate physical guidance | 3 times per minute | 3 out of 6 times | by: (6 hours) |
| Verbalize how anger is expressed. | -with minimal physical guidance | 5 times per minute | __ out of __ times | by: (__ hours) |
| Improve and change behavior to express anger and conflict in an assertive manner. | -with ___% physical guidance | 1 time per hour | 4 consecutive trials out of 8 | by: (1 day) |
| | -with tactile cues | 3 times per hour | 12 consecutive trials out of 15 | by: (3 days) |
| Discuss the advantages and disadvantages of assertive behavior. | -with a demonstration | 5 times per hour | __ consecutive trials out of __ | by: (__ days) |
| Verbalize how assertive behavior relates to communication and socialization. | -with less than 5 verbal prompts | 6 consecutive times per hour | 20% of the time | by: (1 week) |
| | -with less than 3 verbal prompts | 2 times per day | 50% of the time | by: (3 weeks) |
| Report how assertive behavior relates to social skill training. | -with 1 verbal prompt | 3 times per day | ___% of the time | by: (1 month) |
| Recognize and report the relationship between assertion, self-awareness and self-esteem. | -with maximum assistance | 6 times per day | | by: (6 weeks) |
| | -with moderate assistance | 1 time per week | | by: (8 weeks) |
| **Friendships/Relationships.** The client will: | -with minimum assistance | 3 times per week | | by: (3 months) |
| | -with ___% assistance | 8 times per week | | by: (__ months) |
| Define friendship/relationship. | -in the therapy setting | 1 time per month | | |
| Discuss difference between friend, acquaintance, and primary caregiver/family member. | -in the home setting | 3 times per month | | |
| | -independently | 6 times per month | | |
| Identify expectations of a friendship/relationship. | | | | |
| Identify components of a friendship/relationship. | | | | |

Table 10-1 (Continued)

| Social Interaction Skills | **Objective** | | | |
|---|---|---|---|---|
| **Behavioral Task** | **Condition of Performance** | **Frequency or Duration** | **Criteria for Moving to the Next Level of Performance** | **Time Frame** |
| Identify people who are friends. | -with maximum physical guidance | 1 time per minute | 1 out of 3 times | by: (1 hour) |
| Differentiate between acceptable and non-acceptable affection. | -with moderate physical guidance | 3 times per minute | 3 out of 6 times | by: (6 hours) |
| | -with minimal physical guidance | 5 times per minute | __ out of __ times | by: (__ hours) |
| Recognize when to display affection. | -with ___% physical guidance | 1 time per hour | 4 consecutive trials out of 8 | by: (1 day) |
| Display affection to friends and significant others. | -with tactile cues | 3 times per hour | 12 consecutive trials out of 15 | by: (3 days) |
| Identify responsibilities of a friendship/relationship. | -with a demonstration | 5 times per hour | __ consecutive trials out of __ | by: (__ days) |
| | -with less than 5 verbal prompts | 6 consecutive times per hour | 20% of the time | by: (1 week) |
| Verbalize activities that help a friendship continue to grow and develop. | -with less than 3 verbal prompts | 2 times per day | 50% of the time | by: (3 weeks) |
| Verbalize meaning of unconditional friendship/relationship. | -with 1 verbal prompt | 3 times per day | ___% of the time | by: (1 month) |
| | -with maximum assistance | 6 times per day | | by: (6 weeks) |
| Identify and verbalize own feelings in a friendship/relationship. | -with moderate assistance | 1 time per week | | by: (8 weeks) |
| Identify and demonstrate how to develop and end a friendship/relationship. | -with minimum assistance | 3 times per week | | by: (3 months) |
| | -with ___% assistance | 8 times per week | | by: (__ months) |
| Identify and demonstrate how to accept the end of a friendship/relationship. | -in the therapy setting | 1 time per month | | |
| Identify and verbalize how to initiate a friendship/relationship. | -in the home setting | 3 times per month | | |
| | -in a community setting | 6 times per month | | |
| Verbalize how to treat others respectfully. | -independently | | | |
| Demonstrate ability to treat others respectfully. | | | | |
| Interact with individuals who are respectful. | | | | |

© SLACK Inc.

## Therapeutic Suggestions

1. Have individuals in the group practice meeting each other for the first time. Share personal information about self and ask one or two questions to the person you have recently met. Share this information about the new friend to the group.

2. Have group members practice introducing themselves to others. Have each member state name, favorite hobby, and shake hands using a firm grip. Differentiate between handshakes: firm, limp, and too firm.

3. Have group members develop personal and professional goals. Write out what is needed to reach these goals. Have group discuss if all goals are realistic or unrealistic and why. Have members verbalize how they can help each other reach their goals.

4. Give many examples of behavior, have the group discuss which examples are courteous or non-courteous. Have the group role play how non-courteous behaviors may become courteous.

5. Give all members sticks of gum. Have each member demonstrate an example of polite and impolite gum chewing.

6. Have a group of six or fewer members practice table manners during meal time. Have each person demonstrate good and poor sitting posture, napkin and utensil use, selecting normal size portions, and chewing with mouth closed. Have each member ask to be excused when finished.

7. Videotape individuals and the group eating a meal and practicing table manners.

8. Go with group members to a restaurant to practice table skills learned in the home or clinic environment. Use new table manners learned and practice dinner conversation by selecting one topic and have each member discuss one aspect of the topic. Provide constructive feedback to all members and reinforce good conversation behavior immediately.

9. Develop a conversation group. When members enter the room have each introduce self, shaking hands with individuals of the group. Practice maintaining eye contact. Pick one topic to be discussed and have each member participate by adding his thoughts, ideas, and knowledge to the chosen topic. Discuss how own communication patterns effect others.

10. Practice speed and tone of conversation. Model the correct speed and tone, having members imitate. Reinforce all correct imitations as they occur. Have all members practice what is considered loud or fast speech then practice correct speed and tones.

11. Demonstrate logical and illogical speech patterns. Have all members verbalize the difference between both. Discuss how illogical and logical speech affects others when conversing.

12. Discuss use of humor in conversation. Tell tasteful jokes and provide feedback to others on timing of laughter. Discuss the choice of laughter for tasteless jokes that are racist, sexist, and vulgar in nature. Discuss the positive and negative effects of choosing not to laugh.

13. Develop an American Sign Language class for conversing with persons who are hearing impaired. After developing basics, pick one topic for all to discuss. Visit a hearing impaired treatment setting to practice conversation skills using American Sign Language.

14. Demonstrate how to converse using the telephone. Have all members practice calling each other. Begin by making up numbers in the phone book. Call information for new numbers not listed. Practice initiating, maintaining, and ending conversations when talking on phone.

15. Develop a personal telephone book for numbers used most often.

16. Provide a charades group to develop, improve and enhance communication skills.

17. To provide experience for direct communication, have each member practice explaining to someone how to put on a coat.

18. Call a rights advocate to speak to the group on individual rights.

19. Begin a humor group. Encourage spontaneous laughter.

20. Have group members role play passive, assertive, and aggressive behaviors using the same scenario for all role plays. Videotape performances and provide feedback. Have members practice assertive behavior three or more times.

21. Develop a friendship group. Have members pair up with individuals who are not personal friends. Have pairs ask questions of each other while practicing active listening. Have each pair introduce their new friends to the group, mentioning three characteristics of the individual.

# Chapter 11

# Money Management

The purpose of this chapter is to identify basic money management skills needed for independent living. Money management involves basic coin and bill recognition, making and receiving correct change, comparative shopping, budgeting, payment for services and bills, and banking.

The knowledge of currency and understanding of its value and worth can be major facilitating factors aiding in the return to community living after extended hospitalization. Money management can mean the difference between residing in a group home and independent living. There are a complex variety of skills needed to successfully use money. The most important is the ability to compute simple mathematics such as counting, adding, and subtracting. There are assistive devices available for the mathe-matically illiterate, such as calculators and computers which may be taught as splinter skills for functioning independently. These skills and assistive devices are useless unless the individual appreciates the relative value and worth of items to be purchased, and can make prudent decisions on how to spend on a limited income. The typical stereotypic view of the chronic psychiatric patient's management of money entails that all expendable income goes toward cigarettes, coffee, and junk food, leaving nothing left for personal hygiene needs or leisure pursuits. This view can be changed if the client is involved in an educational program that identifies meaningful ways of spending income, involving sensible decision-making skills.

*Table 11-1*

| Money Management | Objective | | | |
|---|---|---|---|---|
| **Behavioral Task** | **Condition of Performance** | **Frequency or Duration** | **Criteria for Moving to the Next Level of Performance** | **Time Frame** |
| **Coin Recognition, Counting, and Making Change.** The client will: | -with maximum physical guidance | 1 time per minute | 1 out of 3 times | by: (1 hour) |
| Recognize coins (penny, nickel, dime, quarter, half dollar). | -with moderate physical guidance | 3 times per minute | 3 out of 6 times | by: (6 hours) |
|  | -with minimal physical guidance | 5 times per minute | __ out of __ times | by: (__ hours) |
| Understand the relative value or worth of coins. | -with ___% physical guidance | 1 time per hour | 4 consecutive trials out of 8 | by: (1 day) |
| Understand the purchasing power of coins (what will a dime buy? a quarter?). | -with tactile cues | 3 times per hour | 12 consecutive trials out of 15 | by: (3 days) |
|  | -with a demonstration | 5 times per hour | __ consecutive trials out of __ | by: (__ days) |
| Count change to $.50. | -with less than 5 verbal prompts | 6 consecutive times per hour | 20% of the time | by: (1 week) |
| Count change to $1.00. | -with less than 3 verbal prompts | 2 times per day | 50% of the time | by: (3 weeks) |
| Count change by fives. | -with 1 verbal prompt | 3 times per day | ___% of the time | by: (1 month) |
| Count change by tens. | -with maximum assistance | 6 times per day |  | by: (6 weeks) |
| Count change by 25. | -with moderate assistance | 1 time per week |  | by: (8 weeks) |
| Identify bills ($1.00, $5.00, $10.00, $20.00). | -with minimum assistance | 3 times per week |  | by: (3 months) |
| Count dollar bills to $5.00. | -with ___% assistance | 8 times per week |  | by: (__ months) |
| Count bills to $10.00. | -in the therapy setting | 1 time per month |  |  |
| Count bills to $25.00. | -in the home setting | 3 times per month |  |  |
| Understand the relative value of bills ($5.00 will purchase more than $1.00). | -in a restaurant setting | 6 times per month |  |  |
| Count bills and coins to $5.00. | -in a store |  |  |  |

*Table 11-1 (Continued)*

| Money Management | Objective | | | |
|---|---|---|---|---|
| **Behavioral Task** | **Condition of Performance** | **Frequency or Duration** | **Criteria for Moving to the Next Level of Performance** | **Time Frame** |
| Count bills and coins to $10.00. | -independently | 1 time per minute | 1 out of 3 times | by: (1 hour) |
| Count bills and coins to $25.00. | -with maximum physical guidance | 3 times per minute | 3 out of 6 times | by: (6 hours) |
| Identify correct change from items less than $.50. | -with moderate physical guidance | 5 times per minute | __ out of __ times | by: (__ hours) |
| Identify correct change from items less than $1.00. | -with minimal physical guidance | 1 time per hour | 4 consecutive trials out of 8 | by: (1 day) |
| | -with ___% physical guidance | 3 times per hour | 12 consecutive trials out of 15 | by: (3 days) |
| Identify correct change from items less than $10.00. | -with tactile cues | 5 times per hour | __ consecutive trials out of __ | by: (__ days) |
| Identify correct change from items less than $25.00. | -with a demonstration | 6 consecutive times per hour | 20% of the time | by: (1 week) |
| | -with less than 5 verbal prompts | 2 times per day | 50% of the time | by: (3 weeks) |
| Identify correct change from items less than $50.00. | -with less than 3 verbal prompts | 3 times per day | ___% of the time | by: (1 month) |
| | -with 1 verbal prompt | 6 times per day | | by: (6 weeks) |
| **Shopping.** The client will: | -with maximum assistance | 1 time per week | | by: (8 weeks) |
| Make a shopping list with a $10.00 limit. | -with moderate assistance | 3 times per week | | by: (3 months) |
| Make a shopping list with a $25.00 limit. | -with minimum assistance | 8 times per week | | by: (__ months) |
| Make up a monthly grocery shopping list with a $50.00 limit. | -with ___% assistance | 1 time per month | | |
| Report items that need to be purchased by primary caregiver. | -in the therapy setting | 3 times per month | | |
| | -in the home setting | 6 times per month | | |
| Go to specified store for items needed. | -in a store | | | |
| Follow shopping list while locating items. | -independently | | | |
| Locate item and price in the store. | | | | |

*Table 11-1 (Continued)*

| *Money Management* | | **Objective** | | |
| --- | --- | --- | --- | --- |
| **Behavioral Task** | **Condition of Performance** | **Frequency or Duration** | **Criteria for Moving to the Next Level of Performance** | **Time Frame** |
| Record price on money counter or by hand. | -with maximum physical guidance | 1 time per minute | 1 out of 3 times | by: (1 hour) |
| Identify total price and denomination needed to purchase item to closest dollar. | -with moderate physical guidance | 3 times per minute | 3 out of 6 times | by: (6 hours) |
| | -with minimal physical guidance | 5 times per minute | __ out of __ times | by: (__ hours) |
| Identify items that can be purchased with food stamps if applicable. | -with ___% physical guidance | 1 time per hour | 4 consecutive trials out of 8 | by: (1 day) |
| Ask assistance for finding shopping items when needed. | -with tactile cues | 3 times per hour | 12 consecutive trials out of 15 | by: (3 days) |
| | -with a demonstration | 5 times per hour | __ consecutive trials out of __ | by: (__ days) |
| Take item to be purchased to the cashier. | -with less than 5 verbal prompts | 6 consecutive times per hour | 20% of the time | by: (1 week) |
| Ask the cashier what the total amount of the purchase is. | -with less than 3 verbal prompts | 2 times per day | 50% of the time | by: (3 weeks) |
| Pay the cashier for the item. | -with 1 verbal prompt | 3 times per day | ___% of the time | by: (1 month) |
| Count change received from the cashier for accuracy. | -with maximum assistance | 6 times per day | | by: (6 weeks) |
| Ask for receipt if necessary. | -with moderate assistance | 1 time per week | | by: (8 weeks) |
| | -with minimum assistance | 3 times per week | | by: (3 months) |
| Compare pricing on hygiene items and determine best value. | -with ___% assistance | 8 times per week | | by: (__ months) |
| Compare pricing on grocery items and determine best value. | -in the therapy setting | 1 time per month | | |
| | -in the home setting | 3 times per month | | |
| Compare pricing on clothing and determine best value. | -in a store | 6 times per month | | |
| Shop for monthly personal hygiene needs with $10.00 limit. | -independently | | | |

*Table 11-1 (Continued)*

| Money Management | | Objective | | |
|---|---|---|---|---|
| **Behavioral Task** | **Condition of Performance** | **Frequency or Duration** | **Criteria for Moving to the Next Level of Performance** | **Time Frame** |
| Determine planned meals for a week and grocery shop for the ingredients. | -with maximum physical guidance | 1 time per minute | 1 out of 3 times | by: (1 hour) |
| Keep a list of groceries and personal items that are expended, for future shopping trips. | -with moderate physical guidance | 3 times per minute | 3 out of 6 times | by: (6 hours) |
| | -with minimal physical guidance | 5 times per minute | __ out of __ times | by: (__ hours) |
| **Banking.** | -with ___% physical guidance | 1 time per hour | 4 consecutive trials out of 8 | by: (1 day) |
| **Savings Account.** The client will: | -with tactile cues | 3 times per hour | 12 consecutive trials out of 15 | by: (3 days) |
| Open a savings account at the bank. | -with a demonstration | 5 times per hour | __ consecutive trials out of __ | by: (__ days) |
| Take money and passbook to bank. | -with less than 5 verbal prompts | 6 consecutive times per hour | 20% of the time | by: (1 week) |
| Wait in line appropriately at the bank. | -with less than 3 verbal prompts | 2 times per day | 50% of the time | by: (3 weeks) |
| Tell teller name and show I.D. | -with 1 verbal prompt | 3 times per day | ___% of the time | by: (1 month) |
| Hand teller the passbook. | -with maximum assistance | 6 times per day | | by: (6 weeks) |
| Complete a savings deposit slip. | -with moderate assistance | 1 time per week | | by: (8 weeks) |
| Complete a savings withdrawal slip. | -with minimum assistance | 3 times per week | | by: (3 months) |
| Hand teller money for a deposit or tell teller amount of money to withdraw. | -with ___% assistance | 8 times per week | | by: (__ months) |
| | -in the therapy setting | 1 time per month | | |
| Wait for passbook or money, ask for receipt if applicable. | -in the home setting | 3 times per month | | |
| Put money in wallet or pocket before leaving bank. | -independently | 6 times per month | | |
| Put passbook in safe place following banking transaction. | -in a public setting | | | |

© SLACK Inc.

97

*Table 11-1 (Continued)*

| Money Management | Objective | | | |
|---|---|---|---|---|
| **Behavioral Task** | **Condition of Performance** | **Frequency or Duration** | **Criteria for Moving to the Next Level of Performance** | **Time Frame** |
| Learn how to use a 24-hour automatic banking system. | -with maximum physical guidance | 1 time per minute | 1 out of 3 times | by: (1 hour) |
| | -with moderate physical guidance | 3 times per minute | 3 out of 6 times | by: (6 hours) |
| **Check Cashing.** The client will: | -with minimal physical guidance | 5 times per minute | __ out of __ times | by: (__ hours) |
| Take check to the bank to be cashed. | -with ___% physical guidance | 1 time per hour | 4 consecutive trials out of 8 | by: (1 day) |
| Sign the back of the check to be cashed. | -with tactile cues | 3 times per hour | 12 consecutive trials out of 15 | by: (3 days) |
| | -with a demonstration | 5 times per hour | __ consecutive trials out of __ | by: (__ days) |
| Hand teller personal I.D. and check to be cashed. | -with less than 5 verbal prompts | 6 consecutive times per hour | 20% of the time | by: (1 week) |
| Wait for the money from the cashed check. | -with less than 3 verbal prompts | 2 times per day | 50% of the time | by: (3 weeks) |
| Put money from cashed check in pocket or wallet before leaving the bank. | -with 1 verbal prompt | 3 times per day | ___% of the time | by: (1 month) |
| | -with maximum assistance | 6 times per day | | by: (6 weeks) |
| **Money Order.** The client will: | -with moderate assistance | 1 time per week | | by: (8 weeks) |
| Take enough money to bank to cover money order and service charge. | -with minimum assistance | 3 times per week | | by: (3 months) |
| Indicate to teller the amount of money order needed. | -with ___% assistance | 8 times per week | | by: (__ months) |
| | -in the therapy setting | 1 time per month | | |
| Hand teller the money and service charge. | -in the home setting | 3 times per month | | |
| Wait for money order and change, if any. | -in a restaurant setting | 6 times per month | | |
| Put money order in wallet or pocket before leaving the bank. | -independently | | | |
| **Checking Account.** The client will: | -in a public setting | | | |
| Open checking account. | | | | |

*Table 11-1 (Continued)*

| Money Management | **Objective** | | | |
|---|---|---|---|---|
| **Behavioral Task** | **Condition of Performance** | **Frequency or Duration** | **Criteria for Moving to the Next Level of Performance** | **Time Frame** |
| Complete a checking account deposit slip. | -with maximum physical guidance | 1 time per minute | 1 out of 3 times | by: (1 hour) |
| Deposit paycheck/SSI/SSD in savings or checking account. | -with moderate physical guidance | 3 times per minute | 3 out of 6 times | by: (6 hours) |
| Record checks written in checkbook. | -with minimal physical guidance | 5 times per minute | __ out of __ times | by: (__ hours) |
| Balance checkbook (by calculator or hand). | -with ___% physical guidance | 1 time per hour | 4 consecutive trials out of 8 | by: (1 day) |
| | -with tactile cues | 3 times per hour | 12 consecutive trials out of 15 | by: (3 days) |
| Read and understand balance indicated on bank account statements. | -with a demonstration | 5 times per hour | __ consecutive trials out of __ | by: (__ days) |
| **Bills and Services.** The client will: | -with less than 5 verbal prompts | 6 consecutive times per hour | 20% of the time | by: (1 week) |
| Identify balance on utility bill. | -with less than 3 verbal prompts | 2 times per day | 50% of the time | by: (3 weeks) |
| Identify balance on telephone bill. | -with 1 verbal prompt | 3 times per day | ___% of the time | by: (1 month) |
| Identify the amount and due date for rent. | -with maximum assistance | 6 times per day | | by: (6 weeks) |
| Demonstrate ability to pay a bill prior to the due date (by hand or mail). | -with moderate assistance | 1 time per week | | by: (8 weeks) |
| | -with minimum assistance | 3 times per week | | by: (3 months) |
| Pay weekly bills (cleaning, grocery) with money allocated for this expense. | -with ___% assistance | 8 times per week | | by: (__ months) |
| Pay for daily expenses (bus tickets, lunches, and miscellaneous items) with money allocated for these expenses. | -in the therapy setting | 1 time per month | | |
| | -in the home setting | 3 times per month | | |
| Pay monthly bills (rent, utilities) with money allocated for these expenses. | -in a community setting | 6 times per month | | |
| | -in a store | | | |
| Demonstrate knowledge of how to pay for medical services (insurance, out of pocket). | -independently | | | |

*Table 11-1 (Continued)*

| Money Management | Objective | | | |
|---|---|---|---|---|
| **Behavioral Task** | **Condition of Performance** | **Frequency or Duration** | **Criteria for Moving to the Next Level of Performance** | **Time Frame** |
| Demonstrate knowledge of how to pay for medication (insurance, out of pocket). | -with maximum physical guidance | 1 time per minute | 1 out of 3 times | by: (1 hour) |
| | -with moderate physical guidance | 3 times per minute | 3 out of 6 times | by: (6 hours) |
| Demonstrate knowledge of how to pay for public transportation needs (bus pass, subway, train). | -with minimal physical guidance | 5 times per minute | __ out of __ times | by: (__ hours) |
| | -with ___% physical guidance | 1 time per hour | 4 consecutive trials out of 8 | by: (1 day) |
| Demonstrate knowledge of how to pay for private transportation (car payments, insurance, maintenance). | -with tactile cues | 3 times per hour | 12 consecutive trials out of 15 | by: (3 days) |
| | -with a demonstration | 5 times per hour | __ consecutive trials out of __ | by: (__ days) |
| **Budgeting.** The client will: | -with less than 5 verbal prompts | 6 consecutive times per hour | 20% of the time | by: (1 week) |
| Plan a monthly itemized budget. | -with less than 3 verbal prompts | 2 times per day | 50% of the time | by: (3 weeks) |
| Identify daily personal requirements or needs and determine if there is money available for them (recreation, food, transportation). | -with 1 verbal prompt | 3 times per day | ___% of the time | by: (1 month) |
| | -with maximum assistance | 6 times per day | | by: (6 weeks) |
| Identify weekly personal requirements or needs and determine if there is money available for them (groceries, hygiene products). | -with moderate assistance | 1 time per week | | by: (8 weeks) |
| | -with minimum assistance | 3 times per week | | by: (3 months) |
| Identify monthly bills (rent, utilities) and determine if there is money available to cover these expenses. | -with ___% assistance | 8 times per week | | by: (__ months) |
| | -in the therapy setting | 1 time per month | | |
| Compare rental unit pricing and determine personal affordability. | -in the home setting | 3 times per month | | |
| | -in a community setting | 6 times per month | | |
| | -independently | | | |

## Therapeutic Suggestions

1. Use empty containers from fast food restaurants and have the client purchase the items using the correct amount of money. Have him check to see if he received the correct change. Have a client sell the item to the purchaser and make correct change.

2. Teach the client how to use a money counter identifying the "ones," "tens," and "hundreds" columns.

3. Go shopping with the client using the money counter.

4. Teach the client how to use a calculator.

5. Go shopping with the client using the calculator to determine the amount of items.

6. Teach the client how to determine the tax on an item so that the correct amount of money will be available for purchase.

7. Use commonly purchased personal hygiene items such as soap, shampoo, and toilet tissue, and simulate selling and purchasing the items making and receiving correct change.

8. Identify which price tags are more or less expensive.

9. Identify which costs more ("Price is Right" technique), a radio or groceries for one month.

10. Go shopping at the grocery store and have the client locate 25 items, and determine the total cost to the nearest dollar of all items (use a money counter or calculator).

11. Given a bill, have the client identify the amount due and the due date. Have him identify when the bill should be mailed to be received by the due date.

12. Practice filling out banking forms.

13. Practice maintaining a checkbook ledger.

14. When looking at price tags, identify what items $5 will purchase.

15. When looking at price tags, identify what items $10 will purchase.

16. Compare two price tags and determine which is more expensive.

17. In the group, practice the correct way to interact with store personnel and cashiers.

18. Using the client's monthly expendable income, determine how much money can be spent on recreation, food, and clothing.

19. Have the client develop a monthly budget and see if he can follow it for one month. Modify according to the client's ability to comply.

20. Have the client look at newspaper flyers and determine which store in town has the best buys on clothing and groceries.

21. Have the client look in the newspaper to determine how much leisure activities cost (movies, bowling, dining, golfing, etc.). Look for comparative bargains for these activities.

# Chapter 12

# Community Mobility

The purpose of this chapter is to provide goals and objectives related to assisting the client in accessing the environment through community travel. To work, socialize, and live as independently as possible requires skills that some individuals may not have in their repertoire. Training programs which provide clients with skills and opportunities to practice components of community mobility are important to increase independence. The area of community mobility is large and encompassing including areas of: walking and bike riding; map reading, taxi, bus, train, subway, and airplane travel; and driving and riding in a car.

*Table 12-1*

| Community Mobility | Objective | | | |
|---|---|---|---|---|
| **Behavioral Task** | **Condition of Performance** | **Frequency or Duration** | **Criteria for Moving to the Next Level of Performance** | **Time Frame** |
| **Walking.** The client will: | -with maximum physical guidance | 1 time per minute | 1 out of 3 times | by: (1 hour) |
| Recognize differences between comfortable and uncomfortable shoes. | -with moderate physical guidance | 3 times per minute | 3 out of 6 times | by: (6 hours) |
| Put on and tie or fasten shoes. | -with minimal physical guidance | 5 times per minute | __ out of __ times | by: (__ hours) |
| Practice and perform breathing techniques. | -with ___% physical guidance | 1 time per hour | 4 consecutive trials out of 8 | by: (1 day) |
| Breathe without difficulty when walking. | -with tactile cues | 3 times per hour | 12 consecutive trials out of 15 | by: (3 days) |
| Walk on correct side of road. | -with a demonstration | 5 times per hour | __ consecutive trials out of __ | by: (__ days) |
| Choose bright/light/reflective clothing when walking at night. | -with less than 5 verbal prompts | 6 consecutive times per hour | 20% of the time | by: (1 week) |
| Walk ___ blocks. | -with less than 3 verbal prompts | 2 times per day | 50% of the time | by: (3 weeks) |
| Plan and take rest breaks. | -with 1 verbal prompt | 3 times per day | ___% of the time | by: (1 month) |
| Walk one mile. | -with maximum assistance | 6 times per day | | by: (6 weeks) |
| Walk with assistive device. | -with moderate assistance | 1 time per week | | by: (8 weeks) |
| Walk to planned destination with assistive device. | -with minimum assistance | 3 times per week | | by: (3 months) |
| Use handrail. | -with ___% assistance | 8 times per week | | by: (__ months) |
| Walk stairs while using a handrail. | -in the therapy setting | 1 time per month | | |
| Walk steep inclines. | -in a community setting | 3 times per month | | |
| Stop and look for traffic before crossing street. | -independently | 6 times per month | | |
| | -correctly | | | |
| | -safely | | | |

© SLACK Inc.

*Table 12-1 (Continued)*

| Community Mobility | Objective | | | |
|---|---|---|---|---|
| **Behavioral Task** | **Condition of Performance** | **Frequency or Duration** | **Criteria for Moving to the Next Level of Performance** | **Time Frame** |
| Recognize and follow walk and do not walk signals/symbols. | -with maximum physical guidance | 1 time per minute | 1 out of 3 times | by: (1 hour) |
| Recognize and use crosswalks. | -with moderate physical guidance | 3 times per minute | 3 out of 6 times | by: (6 hours) |
| Recognize and follow road signs/symbols. | -with minimal physical guidance | 5 times per minute | __ out of __ times | by: (__ hours) |
| Recognize and follow traffic signals. | -with ___% physical guidance | 1 time per hour | 4 consecutive trials out of 8 | by: (1 day) |
| Report or produce living address when asked. | -with tactile cues | 3 times per hour | 12 consecutive trials out of 15 | by: (3 days) |
| Report planned destination when asked. | -with a demonstration | 5 times per hour | __ consecutive trials out of __ | by: (__ days) |
| Walk to planned destination. | -with less than 5 verbal prompts | 6 consecutive times per hour | 20% of the time | by: (1 week) |
| | -with less than 3 verbal prompts | 2 times per day | 50% of the time | by: (3 weeks) |
| **Bicycling.** The client will: | -with 1 verbal prompt | 3 times per day | ___% of the time | by: (1 month) |
| Recognize bicycle lane. | -with maximum assistance | 6 times per day | | by: (6 weeks) |
| Wear proper clothing, head gear, and foot attire. | -with moderate assistance | 1 time per week | | by: (8 weeks) |
| Recognize and use bike signals. | -with minimum assistance | 3 times per week | | by: (3 months) |
| Bicycle on two- or three-wheel bike. | -with ___% assistance | 8 times per week | | by: (__ months) |
| Shift bicycle gears. | -in the therapy setting | 1 time per month | | |
| Bicycle in straight line. | -in a community setting | 3 times per month | | |
| Use brakes. | -independently | 6 times per month | | |
| Bicycle on correct side of road. | -correctly | | | |
| Bicycle up and down steep inclines. | -safely | | | |

© SLACK Inc.

*Table 12-1 (Continued)*

| Community Mobility | Objective | | | |
|---|---|---|---|---|
| **Behavioral Task** | **Condition of Performance** | **Frequency or Duration** | **Criteria for Moving to the Next Level of Performance** | **Time Frame** |
| Turn corners correctly. | -with maximum physical guidance | 1 time per minute | 1 out of 3 times | by: (1 hour) |
| Bike to planned destination. | -with moderate physical guidance | 3 times per minute | 3 out of 6 times | by: (6 hours) |
| **Map Reading.** The client will: | -with minimal physical guidance | 5 times per minute | __ out of __ times | by: (__ hours) |
| Understand terms North, South, East, and West. | -with ___% physical guidance | 1 time per hour | 4 consecutive trials out of 8 | by: (1 day) |
| Point out North, South, East, and West on map. | -with tactile cues | 3 times per hour | 12 consecutive trials out of 15 | by: (3 days) |
| Recognize scale of miles on map. | -with a demonstration | 5 times per hour | __ consecutive trials out of __ | by: (__ days) |
| Measure travel distance on map giving destinations. | -with less than 5 verbal prompts | 6 consecutive times per hour | 20% of the time | by: (1 week) |
| Locate specified streets on travel map. | -with less than 3 verbal prompts | 2 times per day | 50% of the time | by: (3 weeks) |
| Locate parks on travel map. | -with 1 verbal prompt | 3 times per day | ___% of the time | by: (1 month) |
| Locate hospital on travel map. | -with maximum assistance | 6 times per day | | by: (6 weeks) |
| Locate highways on travel map. | -with moderate assistance | 1 time per week | | by: (8 weeks) |
| Recognize paved highway, dirt road, and gravel road on travel map. | -with minimum assistance | 3 times per week | | by: (3 months) |
| | -with ___% assistance | 8 times per week | | by: (__ months) |
| Recognize end of county line on travel map. | -in the therapy setting | 1 time per month | | |
| **Time Usage.** The client will: | -in a community setting | 3 times per month | | |
| Recognize timetable or schedule for bus travel. | -independently | 6 times per month | | |
| | -correctly | | | |
| Verbalize twelve numbers and other parts on face of watch. | -safely | | | |

© SLACK Inc.

*Table 12-1 (Continued)*

| Community Mobility | Objective | | | |
|---|---|---|---|---|
| **Behavioral Task** | **Condition of Performance** | **Frequency or Duration** | **Criteria for Moving to the Next Level of Performance** | **Time Frame** |
| Identify and tell time on clock/watch. | -with maximum physical guidance | 1 time per minute | 1 out of 3 times | by: (1 hour) |
| Set clock correctly when given time. | -with moderate physical guidance | 3 times per minute | 3 out of 6 times | by: (6 hours) |
| **Bus.** The client will: | -with minimal physical guidance | 5 times per minute | __ out of __ times | by: (__ hours) |
| Recognize timetables on bus schedule. | -with ___% physical guidance | 1 time per hour | 4 consecutive trials out of 8 | by: (1 day) |
| Identify arrival and departure columns. | -with tactile cues | 3 times per hour | 12 consecutive trials out of 15 | by: (3 days) |
| Identify departure and arrival times given planned destination. | -with a demonstration | 5 times per hour | __ consecutive trials out of __ | by: (__ days) |
| Recognize and ask for bus transfer slips. | -with less than 5 verbal prompts | 6 consecutive times per hour | 20% of the time | by: (1 week) |
| Transfer buses given planned destination. | -with less than 3 verbal prompts | 2 times per day | 50% of the time | by: (3 weeks) |
| Recognize and purchase bus token or bus pass. | -with 1 verbal prompt | 3 times per day | ___% of the time | by: (1 month) |
| | -with maximum assistance | 6 times per day | | by: (6 weeks) |
| Identify and deposit exact change or token to ride bus. | -with moderate assistance | 1 time per week | | by: (8 weeks) |
| Give bus pass to driver. | -with minimum assistance | 3 times per week | | by: (3 months) |
| | -with ___% assistance | 8 times per week | | by: (__ months) |
| Deposit correct change or token in slot. | -in the therapy setting | 1 time per month | | |
| Seat self on bus or stand if no seat is available. | -in a community setting | 3 times per month | | |
| Forfeit seat for blind or physically handicapped person. | -independently | 6 times per month | | |
| | -correctly | | | |
| Press designated area to signal driver to stop. | -safely | | | |

*Table 12-1 (Continued)*

| Community Mobility | | Objective | | |
|---|---|---|---|---|
| **Behavioral Task** | **Condition of Performance** | **Frequency or Duration** | **Criteria for Moving to the Next Level of Performance** | **Time Frame** |
| Refrain from eating, drinking, or smoking. | -with maximum physical guidance | 1 time per minute | 1 out of 3 times | by: (1 hour) |
| Follow all rules when riding bus. | -with moderate physical guidance | 3 times per minute | 3 out of 6 times | by: (6 hours) |
| Ride bus given planned destination. | -with minimal physical guidance | 5 times per minute | __ out of __ times | by: (__ hours) |
| Ride bus planning own destination. | -with ___% physical guidance | 1 time per hour | 4 consecutive trials out of 8 | by: (1 day) |
| Ride bus alone. | -with tactile cues | 3 times per hour | 12 consecutive trials out of 15 | by: (3 days) |
| **Subway.** The client will: | -with a demonstration | 5 times per hour | __ consecutive trials out of __ | by: (__ days) |
| Recognize subway time schedule. | -with less than 5 verbal prompts | 6 consecutive times per hour | 20% of the time | by: (1 week) |
| Recognize and purchase subway token. | -with less than 3 verbal prompts | 2 times per day | 50% of the time | by: (3 weeks) |
| Transfer subway routes given planned destination. | -with 1 verbal prompt | 3 times per day | ___% of the time | by: (1 month) |
| Seat self on subway or stand if seat is unavailable. | -with maximum assistance | 6 times per day | | by: (6 weeks) |
| | -with moderate assistance | 1 time per week | | by: (8 weeks) |
| Exit subway after reaching destination. | -with minimum assistance | 3 times per week | | by: (3 months) |
| Ride subway given planned destination. | -with ___% assistance | 8 times per week | | by: (__ months) |
| Ride subway alone. | -in the therapy setting | 1 time per month | | |
| **Taxi.** The client will: | -in a community setting | 3 times per month | | |
| Use phone book to locate number of taxi company. | -independently | 6 times per month | | |
| | -correctly | | | |
| Reporting address, request taxi service and ask for amount of money needed for service. | -safely | | | |

© SLACK Inc.

*Table 12-1 (Continued)*

| Community Mobility | | Objective | | |
|---|---|---|---|---|
| **Behavioral Task** | **Condition of Performance** | **Frequency or Duration** | **Criteria for Moving to the Next Level of Performance** | **Time Frame** |
| Sit in back seat of taxi. | -with maximum physical guidance | 1 time per minute | 1 out of 3 times | by: (1 hour) |
| Pay correct fare to taxi driver. | -with moderate physical guidance | 3 times per minute | 3 out of 6 times | by: (6 hours) |
| Tip taxi driver. | -with minimal physical guidance | 5 times per minute | __ out of __ times | by: (__ hours) |
| **Train.** The client will: | -with ___% physical guidance | 1 time per hour | 4 consecutive trials out of 8 | by: (1 day) |
| Identify location of train station. | -with tactile cues | 3 times per hour | 12 consecutive trials out of 15 | by: (3 days) |
| Recognize timetables for train schedules. | -with a demonstration | 5 times per hour | __ consecutive trials out of __ | by: (__ days) |
| Identify departure and arrival times given planned destination. | -with less than 5 verbal prompts | 6 consecutive times per hour | 20% of the time | by: (1 week) |
| | -with less than 3 verbal prompts | 2 times per day | 50% of the time | by: (3 weeks) |
| Eat, drink, and smoke in designated areas. | -with 1 verbal prompt | 3 times per day | ___% of the time | by: (1 month) |
| Plan destination, purchase ticket, and ride train. | -with maximum assistance | 6 times per day | | by: (6 weeks) |
| **Airplane.** The client will: | -with moderate assistance | 1 time per week | | by: (8 weeks) |
| Identify location of airport. | -with minimum assistance | 3 times per week | | by: (3 months) |
| Visit airport. | -with ___% assistance | 8 times per week | | by: (__ months) |
| Identify departure and arrival times of desired carrier. | -in the therapy setting | 1 time per month | | |
| Purchase ticket. | -in a community setting | 3 times per month | | |
| Eat, drink, and smoke in designated areas. | -independently | 6 times per month | | |
| Label luggage with name and address. | -correctly | | | |
| Answer security questions on packed luggage. | -safely | | | |

© SLACK Inc.

*Table 12-1 (Continued)*

| *Community Mobility* | **Objective** | | | |
|---|---|---|---|---|
| **Behavioral Task** | **Condition of Performance** | **Frequency or Duration** | **Criteria for Moving to the Next Level of Performance** | **Time Frame** |
| Give suitcase to airline personnel. | -with maximum physical guidance | 1 time per minute | 1 out of 3 times | by: (1 hour) |
| Go through security checkpoint. | -with moderate physical guidance | 3 times per minute | 3 out of 6 times | by: (6 hours) |
| Find seat matching ticket number. | -with minimal physical guidance | 5 times per minute | __ out of __ times | by: (__ hours) |
| Place carry-on luggage in designated compartment. | -with ___% physical guidance | 1 time per hour | 4 consecutive trials out of 8 | by: (1 day) |
| Fasten seat belt. | -with tactile cues | 3 times per hour | 12 consecutive trials out of 15 | by: (3 days) |
| | -with a demonstration | 5 times per hour | __ consecutive trials out of __ | by: (__ days) |
| Unfasten seat belt when airline personnel allow. | -with less than 5 verbal prompts | 6 consecutive times per hour | 20% of the time | by: (1 week) |
| Leave plane. | -with less than 3 verbal prompts | 2 times per day | 50% of the time | by: (3 weeks) |
| Complete customs process. | -with 1 verbal prompt | 3 times per day | ___% of the time | by: (1 month) |
| Go to luggage area and find luggage. | -with maximum assistance | 6 times per day | | by: (6 weeks) |
| Leave airport. | -with moderate assistance | 1 time per week | | by: (8 weeks) |
| **Car.** The client will: | -with minimum assistance | 3 times per week | | by: (3 months) |
| Fasten seat belt. | -with ___% assistance | 8 times per week | | by: (__ months) |
| Assist driver with planned destination if needed. | -in the therapy setting | 1 time per month | | |
| Ask to smoke before lighting cigarette. | -in a community setting | 3 times per month | | |
| Attend driver education course. | -correctly | | | |
| Complete driver education course. | -safely | | | |

*Table 12-1 (Continued)*

| Community Mobility | Objective | | | |
|---|---|---|---|---|
| **Behavioral Task** | **Condition of Performance** | **Frequency or Duration** | **Criteria for Moving to the Next Level of Performance** | **Time Frame** |
| Complete driver education test, written and performance. | -with maximum physical guidance | 1 time per minute | 1 out of 3 times | by: (1 hour) |
| | -with moderate physical guidance | 3 times per minute | 3 out of 6 times | by: (6 hours) |
| Obtain driver's license application. | -with minimal physical guidance | 5 times per minute | __ out of __ times | by: (__ hours) |
| Understand words used on application. | -with ___% physical guidance | 1 time per hour | 4 consecutive trials out of 8 | by: (1 day) |
| Complete application. | -with tactile cues | 3 times per hour | 12 consecutive trials out of 15 | by: (3 days) |
| Verbalize and practice road safety. | -with a demonstration | 5 times per hour | __ consecutive trials out of __ | by: (__ days) |
| Use parking meter. | -with less than 5 verbal prompts | 6 consecutive times per hour | 20% of the time | by: (1 week) |
| Purchase car. | -with less than 3 verbal prompts | 2 times per day | 50% of the time | by: (3 weeks) |
| Purchase license plate. | -with 1 verbal prompt | 3 times per day | ___% of the time | by: (1 month) |
| Purchase insurance. | -with maximum assistance | 6 times per day | | by: (6 weeks) |
| | -with moderate assistance | 1 time per week | | by: (8 weeks) |
| | -with minimum assistance | 3 times per week | | by: (3 months) |
| | -with ___% assistance | 8 times per week | | by: (__ months) |
| | -in the therapy setting | 1 time per month | | |
| | -in a community setting | 3 times per month | | |
| | -independently | 6 times per month | | |
| | -correctly | | | |
| | -safely | | | |

## Therapeutic Suggestions

1. Group together a variety of shoes with different shapes, sizes, and heel levels. Have client place all shoes in a row going from most comfortable to the least comfortable walking shoe.

2. In group settings, practice breathing techniques for walking and biking, modeling behavior. Demonstrate difference between deep breathing, shallow breathing, and relaxed breathing.

3. Have clients each blow up a balloon, slowly letting the air out. Relate the balloon activity to the bodily function of breathing. Also use the balloon to develop and increase breathing capacity.

4. Mix a large variety of clothing in a pile. Have the clients pick out clothes they would wear if walking or riding a bike at dusk or dark.

5. Develop a walking course, and give clients a map. Include areas with stairs and steep inclines. Have area labelled on map where forward and backward walking are required.

6. Place road signs around the clinic or treatment environment. Walk around the setting asking client or group what each sign says and means, where the sign is most often see, and what is required to follow the sign.

7. Have all clients operate stationary bike, bike with training wheels, and tandem bicycle. After all succeed, have them incorporate bike signals when riding.

8. Give each client a map. Ask questions regarding location of North, South, East, and West. Ask client to use map scale measuring the number of miles from two given destinations. Have him draw the travel route he would most like to use. Each week select a specific person's route, having him lead the group to the planned destination.

9. Visit bus station, having each client pick up a variety of schedules. Orient client to departure and arrival columns. Ask simulated questions on if bus leaves _____ when will it arrive at _____.

10. Visit train station, having client pick up a variety of schedules. Orient client to departure and arrival columns. Ask simulated questions on if train leaves _____ when will it arrive at _____.

11. Have each client pick a route to travel on bus. Each week have group travel one of the selected places.

12. Separate group into pairs; have each pair select a bus route to travel. Have each pair go independently and discuss travel activity as a group.

13. Visit train station picking a destination all group members would like to visit. Have each member purchase ticket separately and leave as a group to planned destination.

14. Have group practice completing driver's application. Question members regarding words not recognized and any unclear meanings of questions. Ask group members to answer each other's questions; only clarify when necessary.

15. Have group verbalize situations when driving is not appropriate and alternative transportation available in these instances, e.g., drinking, medication usage, and poor eyesight and coordination may lead individual to use bus system, train, or taxi service.

16. Practice looking in the telephone book and calling bus, train, airport, subway, and taxi services for price of tickets given planned destination.

17. Visit used car lots looking at cost of vehicles. Price insurance payments to determine monthly budget for purchasing a car.

112

# Chapter 13

# Health-Related Behaviors

The purpose of this chapter is to provide an overview of behaviors necessary for individuals to become independent in the area of health. In order to live in an independent or semi-independent community setting, knowledge in the area of health skills is important for survival. Health-related behaviors can be divided into categories of skin, eye and ear care, office appointments, dental care, medication, personal health, diet and exercise, stress management, proper body mechanics, and substance education.

The areas which comprise health-related behaviors are important in that they directly relate to the field of mental health. For example, when an individual experiences emotional difficulties, the area that may need attention is medication. Individuals who have received education and training regarding medication may prevent a psychiatric relapse from occurring by being aware of the signs and symptoms of their condition. They may then seek a medication review and an adjustment could be made, thus preventing the need for hospitalization. The clinician or health care professional needs to be aware of the areas of health-related behaviors that the individuals need to strengthen in order to help them reach the highest level of independence possible.

*Table 13-1*

| Health-Related Behaviors | Objective | | | |
|---|---|---|---|---|
| **Behavioral Task** | **Condition of Performance** | **Frequency or Duration** | **Criteria for Moving to the Next Level of Performance** | **Time Frame** |
| **Skin Care.** The client will: | | | | |
| Recognize difference between healthy and unhealthy skin. | -with maximum physical guidance | 1 time per minute | 1 out of 3 times | by: (1 hour) |
| | -with moderate physical guidance | 3 times per minute | 3 out of 6 times | by: (6 hours) |
| Recognize difference between dry and oily skin. | -with minimal physical guidance | 5 times per minute | __ out of __ times | by: (__ hours) |
| Recognize skin chapped from weather conditions. | -with ___% physical guidance | 1 time per hour | 4 consecutive trials out of 8 | by: (1 day) |
| | -with tactile cues | 3 times per hour | 12 consecutive trials out of 15 | by: (3 days) |
| Check skin for irregularities. | -with a demonstration | 5 times per hour | __ consecutive trials out of __ | by: (__ days) |
| Apply lotion/ointment/powder to affected areas as needed. | -with less than 3 verbal prompts | 6 consecutive times per hour | 20% of the time | by: (1 week) |
| Apply ointment to chapped lips. | -with 1 verbal prompt | 2 times per day | 50% of the time | by: (3 weeks) |
| Purchase over-the-counter medication for specific problems. | -with maximum assistance | 3 times per day | ___% of the time | by: (1 month) |
| | -with moderate assistance | 6 times per day | | by: (6 weeks) |
| Recognize and treat callouses, ingrown nails, and warts on hand. | -with minimum assistance | 1 time per week | | by: (8 weeks) |
| Recognize and treat a corn, callous, bunion, wart, rash, or athletes foot on feet. | -with ___% assistance | 3 times per week | | by: (3 months) |
| | -in the therapy setting | 8 times per week | | by: (__ months) |
| Wash hands after applying material/ointments. | -in the home setting | 1 time per month | | |
| Apply moleskin, bandages, and gauze. | -independently | 3 times per month | | |
| Wear protective clothing in adverse weather. | -correctly | 6 times per month | | |
| Recognize, prevent, and treat skin for photosensitivity due to psychotropics. | -accurately | | | |

*Table 13-1 (Continued)*

| Health-Related Behaviors | Objective | | | |
|---|---|---|---|---|
| **Behavioral Task** | **Condition of Performance** | **Frequency or Duration** | **Criteria for Moving to the Next Level of Performance** | **Time Frame** |
| **Eye and Ear Care.** The client will: | | | | |
| Recognize clear and unclear vision. | -with maximum physical guidance | 1 time per minute | 1 out of 3 times | by: (1 hour) |
| Recognize and identify color blindness. | -with moderate physical guidance | 3 times per minute | 3 out of 6 times | by: (6 hours) |
| Report when vision problems occur. | -with minimal physical guidance | 5 times per minute | __ out of __ times | by: (__ hours) |
| Schedule eye appointments and arrive on time. | -with ___% physical guidance | 1 time per hour | 4 consecutive trials out of 8 | by: (1 day) |
| | -with tactile cues | 3 times per hour | 12 consecutive trials out of 15 | by: (3 days) |
| Follow ophthalmologist's or optometrist's instructions. | -with a demonstration | 5 times per hour | __ consecutive trials out of __ | by: (__ days) |
| Wear and clean glasses regularly. | -with less than 3 verbal prompts | 6 consecutive times per hour | 20% of the time | by: (1 week) |
| Store glasses in proper position. | -with 1 verbal prompt | 2 times per day | 50% of the time | by: (3 weeks) |
| Wear and care for contact lenses. | -with maximum assistance | 3 times per day | ___% of the time | by: (1 month) |
| Purchase proper lens care materials. | -with moderate assistance | 6 times per day | | by: (6 weeks) |
| Wear ear protectors when in loud environment. | -with minimum assistance | 1 time per week | | by: (8 weeks) |
| | -with ___% assistance | 3 times per week | | by: (3 months) |
| Clean and care for ears. | -in the therapy setting | 8 times per week | | by: (__ months) |
| Apply ear drops when needed. | -in the home setting | 1 time per month | | |
| Report signs and symptoms of ear problems to physician. | -independently | 3 times per month | | |
| **Office Appointments.** The client will: | -correctly | 6 times per month | | |
| Identify physician needed for appointment. | -accurately | | | |

*Table 13-1 (Continued)*

| Health-Related Behaviors | Objective | | | |
|---|---|---|---|---|
| **Behavioral Task** | **Condition of Performance** | **Frequency or Duration** | **Criteria for Moving to the Next Level of Performance** | **Time Frame** |
| Call desired physician's office or health department to schedule appointment. | -with maximum physical guidance | 1 time per minute | 1 out of 3 times | by: (1 hour) |
| | -with moderate physical guidance | 3 times per minute | 3 out of 6 times | by: (6 hours) |
| Arrive on time to appointments and bring insurance card/number. | -with minimal physical guidance | 5 times per minute | __ out of __ times | by: (__ hours) |
| Fill out health care insurance forms. | -with ___% physical guidance | 1 time per hour | 4 consecutive trials out of 8 | by: (1 day) |
| Report signs and symptoms to physician/ nurse. | -with tactile cues | 3 times per hour | 12 consecutive trials out of 15 | by: (3 days) |
| | -with a demonstration | 5 times per hour | __ consecutive trials out of __ | by: (__ days) |
| Answer health-related questions. | -with less than 5 verbal prompts | 6 consecutive times per hour | 20% of the time | by: (1 week) |
| Cooperate with blood work/x-ray/physical examination procedures. | -with less than 3 verbal prompts | 2 times per day | 50% of the time | by: (3 weeks) |
| Cooperate, repeat, and follow doctor's orders. | -with 1 verbal prompt | 3 times per day | ___% of the time | by: (1 month) |
| Call physician's office to report abnormal signs and symptoms of medication. | -with maximum assistance | 6 times per day | | by: (6 weeks) |
| | -with moderate assistance | 1 time per week | | by: (8 weeks) |
| **Dental Care.** The client will: | -with minimum assistance | 3 times per week | | by: (3 months) |
| Recognize and identify healthy and unhealthy teeth. | -with ___% assistance | 8 times per week | | by: (__ months) |
| Verbalize what causes teeth staining and how to prevent it. | -in the therapy setting | 1 time per month | | |
| | -in the home setting | 3 times per month | | |
| Brush and floss teeth, brush tongue, use mouthwash. | -independently | 6 times per month | | |
| Report bleeding gums. | -correctly | | | |
| Replace old and worn dental items. | -accurately | | | |

*Table 13-1 (Continued)*

| *Health-Related Behaviors* | | **Objective** | | |
|---|---|---|---|---|
| **Behavioral Task** | **Condition of Performance** | **Frequency or Duration** | **Criteria for Moving to the Next Level of Performance** | **Time Frame** |
| Report when out of supplies. | -with maximum physical guidance | 1 time per minute | 1 out of 3 times | by: (1 hour) |
| Report dental pain and sensitivity to hot/cold/sugary items. | -with moderate physical guidance | 3 times per minute | 3 out of 6 times | by: (6 hours) |
| Wear dentures or partial plates. | -with minimal physical guidance | 5 times per minute | __ out of __ times | by: (__ hours) |
| Care for dentures. | -with ___% physical guidance | 1 time per hour | 4 consecutive trials out of 8 | by: (1 day) |
| Use denture gripping agent. | -with tactile cues | 3 times per hour | 12 consecutive trials out of 15 | by: (3 days) |
| | -with a demonstration | 5 times per hour | __ consecutive trials out of __ | by: (__ days) |
| **Medication.** The client will: | -with less than 5 verbal prompts | 6 consecutive times per hour | 20% of the time | by: (1 week) |
| Verbalize and understand why medication is necessary. | -with less than 3 verbal prompts | 2 times per day | 50% of the time | by: (3 weeks) |
| Be aware of times to take medication and follow through. | -with 1 verbal prompt | 3 times per day | ___% of the time | by: (1 month) |
| | -with maximum assistance | 6 times per day | | by: (6 weeks) |
| Go to primary caregiver to request medication. | -with moderate assistance | 1 time per week | | by: (8 weeks) |
| Measure required amount of medication. | -with minimum assistance | 3 times per week | | by: (3 months) |
| Swallow medication. | -with ___% assistance | 8 times per week | | by: (__ months) |
| Read and follow medication dosage on bottle. | -in the therapy setting | 1 time per month | | |
| Refill medication before empty. | -in the home setting | 3 times per month | | |
| Recognize different forms of medication. | -independently | 6 times per month | | |
| Understand and verbalize the effects of drugs and alcohol when mixed with medication. | -correctly | | | |
| | -accurately | | | |

*Table 13-1 (Continued)*

| Health-Related Behaviors | Objective | | | |
|---|---|---|---|---|
| **Behavioral Task** | **Condition of Performance** | **Frequency or Duration** | **Criteria for Moving to the Next Level of Performance** | **Time Frame** |
| Know name of medication taking. | -with maximum physical guidance | 1 time per minute | 1 out of 3 times | by: (1 hour) |
| Report relationship between certain medication and sun sensitivity. | -with moderate physical guidance | 3 times per minute | 3 out of 6 times | by: (6 hours) |
| Use sunscreen when outside. | -with minimal physical guidance | 5 times per minute | __ out of __ times | by: (__ hours) |
| Follow warning signs of medication. | -with ___% physical guidance | 1 time per hour | 4 consecutive trials out of 8 | by: (1 day) |
| Be aware of all possible side effects of medication. | -with tactile cues | 3 times per hour | 12 consecutive trials out of 15 | by: (3 days) |
|  | -with a demonstration | 5 times per hour | __ consecutive trials out of __ | by: (__ days) |
| Report medication side effects to appropriate person. | -with less than 5 verbal prompts | 6 consecutive times per hour | 20% of the time | by: (1 week) |
| Do not take unprescribed medication. | -with less than 3 verbal prompts | 2 times per day | 50% of the time | by: (3 weeks) |
| Pack medication for overnight stays and label clearly. | -with 1 verbal prompt | 3 times per day | ___% of the time | by: (1 month) |
|  | -with maximum assistance | 6 times per day |  | by: (6 weeks) |
| Store medication as directed. | -with moderate assistance | 1 time per week |  | by: (8 weeks) |
| Flush medication when outdated. | -with minimum assistance | 3 times per week |  | by: (3 months) |
| Change medication dosage when indicated by physician. | -with ___% assistance | 8 times per week |  | by: (__ months) |
| Have levels of medication in blood checked regularly. | -in the therapy setting | 1 time per month |  |  |
|  | -in the home setting | 3 times per month |  |  |
| Attend monthly medication review check-ups. | -independently | 6 times per month |  |  |
| Attend and participate in medication classes. | -correctly |  |  |  |
|  | -accurately |  |  |  |

*Table 13-1 (Continued)*

| Health-Related Behaviors | Objective | | | |
|---|---|---|---|---|

| Behavioral Task | Condition of Performance | Frequency or Duration | Criteria for Moving to the Next Level of Performance | Time Frame |
|---|---|---|---|---|
| **Personal Health.** The client will: | | | | |
| Recognize difference between male and female anatomy. | -with maximum physical guidance | 1 time per minute | 1 out of 3 times | by: (1 hour) |
| | -with moderate physical guidance | 3 times per minute | 3 out of 6 times | by: (6 hours) |
| Verbalize the basic maturation process. | -with minimal physical guidance | 5 times per minute | __ out of __ times | by: (__ hours) |
| Recognize steps of menstrual cycle. | -with ___% physical guidance | 1 time per hour | 4 consecutive trials out of 8 | by: (1 day) |
| Verbalize the difference of male and female reproductive systems. | -with tactile cues | 3 times per hour | 12 consecutive trials out of 15 | by: (3 days) |
| Report how sexual intercourse is related to conception. | -with a demonstration | 5 times per hour | __ consecutive trials out of __ | by: (__ days) |
| | -with less than 3 verbal prompts | 6 consecutive times per hour | 20% of the time | by: (1 week) |
| Verbalize psychotropic medications that interfere with erections/ejaculation. | -with 1 verbal prompt | 2 times per day | 50% of the time | by: (3 weeks) |
| Know and verbalize how pregnancy can be prevented. | -with maximum assistance | 3 times per day | ___% of the time | by: (1 month) |
| | -with moderate assistance | 6 times per day | | by: (6 weeks) |
| Verbalize what birth control is. | -with minimum assistance | 1 time per week | | by: (8 weeks) |
| Verbalize what abstinence is. | -with ___% assistance | 3 times per week | | by: (3 months) |
| Identify, report, and explain various methods of male and female birth control. | -in the therapy setting | 8 times per week | | by: (__ months) |
| Recognize effect of psychotropic medication on birth complications. | -in the home setting | 1 time per month | | |
| | -independently | 3 times per month | | |
| Recognize symptoms of pregnancy. | -correctly | 6 times per month | | |
| Verbalize definition of sexually transmitted diseases (STD). | -accurately | | | |

*Table 13-1 (Continued)*

| Health-Related Behaviors | Objective | | | |
|---|---|---|---|---|
| **Behavioral Task** | **Condition of Performance** | **Frequency or Duration** | **Criteria for Moving to the Next Level of Performance** | **Time Frame** |
| Recognize signs and symptoms of STD's. | -with maximum physical guidance | 1 time per minute | 1 out of 3 times | by: (1 hour) |
| Recognize and understand how to prevent STD's from occurring. | -with moderate physical guidance | 3 times per minute | 3 out of 6 times | by: (6 hours) |
| | -with minimal physical guidance | 5 times per minute | __ out of __ times | by: (__ hours) |
| Seek immediate help if recognizing any signs and symptoms of STD's. | -with ___% physical guidance | 1 time per hour | 4 consecutive trials out of 8 | by: (1 day) |
| Verbalize what AIDS is and who is at risk to contract it. | -with tactile cues | 3 times per hour | 12 consecutive trials out of 15 | by: (3 days) |
| | -with a demonstration | 5 times per hour | __ consecutive trials out of __ | by: (__ days) |
| Verbalize how to prevent AIDS from occurring. | -with less than 5 verbal prompts | 6 consecutive times per hour | 20% of the time | by: (1 week) |
| **Diet and Exercise.** The client will: | -with less than 3 verbal prompts | 2 times per day | 50% of the time | by: (3 weeks) |
| Identify appropriate number of each food group to eat per day. | -with 1 verbal prompt | 3 times per day | ___% of the time | by: (1 month) |
| | -with maximum assistance | 6 times per day | | by: (6 weeks) |
| Verbalize relationship between food and good mental health. | -with moderate assistance | 1 time per week | | by: (8 weeks) |
| Identify and recognize the effects of fat, cholesterol, sodium, and sugar to body functioning. | -with minimum assistance | 3 times per week | | by: (3 months) |
| | -with ___% assistance | 8 times per week | | by: (__ months) |
| Identify average portions of each food group. | -in the therapy setting | 1 time per month | | |
| Recognize how smoking leads to disease. | -in the home setting | 3 times per month | | |
| Recognize the effects of caffeine on body functioning. | -independently | 6 times per month | | |
| | -correctly | | | |
| Identify and use different methods to prepare more nutritious meals. | -accurately | | | |

*Table 13-1 (Continued)*

| Health-Related Behaviors | Objective | | | |
|---|---|---|---|---|
| **Behavioral Task** | **Condition of Performance** | **Frequency or Duration** | **Criteria for Moving to the Next Level of Performance** | **Time Frame** |
| Identify ways to substitute ingredients in recipes to decrease fat, cholesterol, sodium, and sugar. | -with maximum physical guidance | 1 time per minute | 1 out of 3 times | by: (1 hour) |
| | -with moderate physical guidance | 3 times per minute | 3 out of 6 times | by: (6 hours) |
| Identify and perform activities that promote good mental health. | -with minimal physical guidance | 5 times per minute | __ out of __ times | by: (__ hours) |
| | -with ___% physical guidance | 1 time per hour | 4 consecutive trials out of 8 | by: (1 day) |
| Recognize relationship between exercise and good mental health. | -with tactile cues | 3 times per hour | 12 consecutive trials out of 15 | by: (3 days) |
| Recognize how to pace self in exercise program. | -with a demonstration | 5 times per hour | __ consecutive trials out of __ | by: (__ days) |
| | -with less than 5 verbal prompts | 6 consecutive times per hour | 20% of the time | by: (1 week) |
| Identify and perform exercises that improve the cardiovascular system. | -with less than 3 verbal prompts | 2 times per day | 50% of the time | by: (3 weeks) |
| Identify and perform exercises to improve musculoskeletal system. | -with 1 verbal prompt | 3 times per day | ___% of the time | by: (1 month) |
| | -with maximum assistance | 6 times per day | | by: (6 weeks) |
| Identify proper ways to exercise. | -with moderate assistance | 1 time per week | | by: (8 weeks) |
| Take pulse at neck and wrist. | -with minimum assistance | 3 times per week | | by: (3 months) |
| Identify and evaluate target heart rate during exercise. | -with ___% assistance | 8 times per week | | by: (__ months) |
| Identify resting heart rate. | -in the therapy setting | 1 time per month | | |
| Recognize signs and symptoms of over-exertion. | -in the home setting | 3 times per month | | |
| | -independently | 6 times per month | | |
| Identify how to improve own exercise level. | -correctly | | | |
| Write and follow diet and exercise plan. | -accurately | | | |

*Table 13-1 (Continued)*

| Health-Related Behaviors | Objective | | | |
|---|---|---|---|---|
| **Behavioral Task** | **Condition of Performance** | **Frequency or Duration** | **Criteria for Moving to the Next Level of Performance** | **Time Frame** |
| Identify proper clothing to wear during exercise. | -with maximum physical guidance | 1 time per minute | 1 out of 3 times | by: (1 hour) |
| Recognize need to drink water. | -with moderate physical guidance | 3 times per minute | 3 out of 6 times | by: (6 hours) |
| | -with minimal physical guidance | 5 times per minute | __ out of __ times | by: (__ hours) |
| **Stress Management.** The client will: | -with ___% physical guidance | 1 time per hour | 4 consecutive trials out of 8 | by: (1 day) |
| Identify relationship between stress and health. | -with tactile cues | 3 times per hour | 12 consecutive trials out of 15 | by: (3 days) |
| Identify causes of stress and how to handle productively. | -with a demonstration | 5 times per hour | __ consecutive trials out of __ | by: (__ days) |
| Recognize signs and symptoms of stress. | -with less than 5 verbal prompts | 6 consecutive times per hour | 20% of the time | by: (1 week) |
| Select and perform options/activities that decrease stress behaviors. | -with less than 3 verbal prompts | 2 times per day | 50% of the time | by: (3 weeks) |
| | -with 1 verbal prompt | 3 times per day | ___% of the time | by: (1 month) |
| Verbalize importance of relaxation. | -with maximum assistance | 6 times per day | | by: (6 weeks) |
| Identify and report sources of relaxation. | -with moderate assistance | 1 time per week | | by: (8 weeks) |
| Listen to relaxation tapes. | -with minimum assistance | 3 times per week | | by: (3 months) |
| Recognize and perform self-relaxation. | -with ___% assistance | 8 times per week | | by: (__ months) |
| Listen to relaxing music. | -in the therapy setting | 1 time per month | | |
| Identify strategies to address stress-related problems. | -in the home setting | 3 times per month | | |
| Know when to seek help for crisis situation. | -independently | 6 times per month | | |
| | -correctly | | | |
| | -accurately | | | |

*Table 13-1 (Continued)*

| Health-Related Behaviors | Objective | | | |
|---|---|---|---|---|
| **Behavioral Task** | **Condition of Performance** | **Frequency or Duration** | **Criteria for Moving to the Next Level of Performance** | **Time Frame** |
| **Body Mechanics.** The client will: | | | | |
| Recognize spine and supporting structures. | -with maximum physical guidance | 1 time per minute | 1 out of 3 times | by: (1 hour) |
| Recognize that there are numerous muscles attached to spine. | -with moderate physical guidance | 3 times per minute | 3 out of 6 times | by: (6 hours) |
| | -with minimal physical guidance | 5 times per minute | __ out of __ times | by: (__ hours) |
| Recognize correct and incorrect body posture. | -with ___% physical guidance | 1 time per hour | 4 consecutive trials out of 8 | by: (1 day) |
| Verbalize and demonstrate correct sitting and standing postures. | -with tactile cues | 3 times per hour | 12 consecutive trials out of 15 | by: (3 days) |
| Verbalize and demonstrate correct sleeping postures. | -with a demonstration | 5 times per hour | __ consecutive trials out of __ | by: (__ days) |
| Practice correct body posture performing daily activities. | -with less than 3 verbal prompts | 6 consecutive times per hour | 20% of the time | by: (1 week) |
| | -with 1 verbal prompt | 2 times per day | 50% of the time | by: (3 weeks) |
| Verbalize three or more causes of back injuries. | -with maximum assistance | 3 times per day | ___% of the time | by: (1 month) |
| | -with moderate assistance | 6 times per day | | by: (6 weeks) |
| Verbalize difference between muscle spasm, back strain, and ruptured disk. | -with minimum assistance | 1 time per week | | by: (8 weeks) |
| Report back injuries to proper health professional. | -with ___% assistance | 3 times per week | | by: (3 months) |
| | -in the therapy setting | 8 times per week | | by: (__ months) |
| Practice proper lifting and moving techniques. | -in the home setting | 1 time per month | | |
| Verbalize ways to adapt environment to prevent back injuries. | -independently | 3 times per month | | |
| Analyze and change living and working environment to reduce and prevent injuries. | -correctly | 6 times per month | | |
| | -accurately | | | |

*Table 13-1 (Continued)*

| Health-Related Behaviors | Objective | | | |
|---|---|---|---|---|
| **Behavioral Task** | **Condition of Performance** | **Frequency or Duration** | **Criteria for Moving to the Next Level of Performance** | **Time Frame** |
| Change habits that increase risk of back injuries. | -with maximum physical guidance | 1 time per minute | 1 out of 3 times | by: (1 hour) |
| Perform back exercises. | -with moderate physical guidance | 3 times per minute | 3 out of 6 times | by: (6 hours) |
| Improve fitness level. | -with minimal physical guidance | 5 times per minute | __ out of __ times | by: (__ hours) |
| Perform six individualized back exercises as prescribed by doctor or other health provider. | -with ___% physical guidance | 1 time per hour | 4 consecutive trials out of 8 | by: (1 day) |
| | -with tactile cues | 3 times per hour | 12 consecutive trials out of 15 | by: (3 days) |
| | -with a demonstration | 5 times per hour | __ consecutive trials out of __ | by: (__ days) |
| **Substance Abuse.** The client will: | -with less than 5 verbal prompts | 6 consecutive times per hour | 20% of the time | by: (1 week) |
| Verbalize risks associated with smoking. | -with less than 3 verbal prompts | 2 times per day | 50% of the time | by: (3 weeks) |
| Learn and demonstrate techniques used to help stop smoking. | -with 1 verbal prompt | 3 times per day | ___% of the time | by: (1 month) |
| Report services provided by American Cancer Society. | -with maximum assistance | 6 times per day | | by: (6 weeks) |
| Stop smoking. | -with moderate assistance | 1 time per week | | by: (8 weeks) |
| Report negative effects of alcohol. | -with minimum assistance | 3 times per week | | by: (3 months) |
| Verbalize danger of drinking alcohol and operating a motor vehicle or machinery. | -with ___% assistance | 8 times per week | | by: (__ months) |
| Verbalize effects of medication mixed with alcohol. | -in the therapy setting | 1 time per month | | |
| | -in the home setting | 3 times per month | | |
| Attend Alcoholics Anonymous meeting. | -independently | 6 times per month | | |
| Report risks associated with overeating. | -correctly | | | |
| | -accurately | | | |

*Table 13-1 (Continued)*

| Health-Related Behaviors | Objective | | | |
|---|---|---|---|---|
| **Behavioral Task** | **Condition of Performance** | **Frequency or Duration** | **Criteria for Moving to the Next Level of Performance** | **Time Frame** |
| Identify and perform alternative activities. | -with maximum physical guidance | 1 time per minute | 1 out of 3 times | by: (1 hour) |
| Follow diet as prescribed by doctor or dietician. | -with moderate physical guidance | 3 times per minute | 3 out of 6 times | by: (6 hours) |
| Attend Overeaters Anonymous meeting. | -with minimal physical guidance | 5 times per minute | __ out of __ times | by: (__ hours) |
| | -with ___% physical guidance | 1 time per hour | 4 consecutive trials out of 8 | by: (1 day) |
| Increase physical activity in relation to food consumption. | -with tactile cues | 3 times per hour | 12 consecutive trials out of 15 | by: (3 days) |
| Verbalize foods/drinks with caffeine in them. | -with a demonstration | 5 times per hour | __ consecutive trials out of __ | by: (__ days) |
| Verbalize effects of caffeine regarding behavior. | -with less than 5 verbal prompts | 6 consecutive times per hour | 20% of the time | by: (1 week) |
| | -with less than 3 verbal prompts | 2 times per day | 50% of the time | by: (3 weeks) |
| Report the effects of caffeine combined with prescription medication. | -with 1 verbal prompt | 3 times per day | ___% of the time | by: (1 month) |
| Increase use of noncaffeinated beverages. | -with maximum assistance | 6 times per day | | by: (6 weeks) |
| Report what water intoxication is. | -with moderate assistance | 1 time per week | | by: (8 weeks) |
| Develop and complete alternative activities to drinking large amounts of water. | -with minimum assistance | 3 times per week | | by: (3 months) |
| | -with ___% assistance | 8 times per week | | by: (__ months) |
| Report difference between legal and illegal drugs. | -in the therapy setting | 1 time per month | | |
| Verbalize negative effects of illegal substances. | -in the home setting | 3 times per month | | |
| | -independently | 6 times per month | | |
| Report negative effects of illegal substances when combined with prescription medication. | -correctly | | | |
| Develop and perform alternative hobbies and activities. | -accurately | | | |

© SLACK Inc.

*Table 13-1 (Continued)*

| Health-Related Behaviors | | | Objective | |
|---|---|---|---|---|
| **Behavioral Task** | **Condition of Performance** | **Frequency or Duration** | **Criteria for Moving to the Next Level of Performance** | **Time Frame** |
| Develop peer relationships with individuals who do not use illegal substances.<br><br>Attend Narcotics Anonymous. | -with maximum physical guidance | 1 time per minute | 1 out of 3 times | by: (1 hour) |
| | -with moderate physical guidance | 3 times per minute | 3 out of 6 times | by: (6 hours) |
| | -with minimal physical guidance | 5 times per minute | __ out of __ times | by: (__ hours) |
| | -with ___% physical guidance | 1 time per hour | 4 consecutive trials out of 8 | by: (1 day) |
| | -with tactile cues | 3 times per hour | 12 consecutive trials out of 15 | by: (3 days) |
| | -with a demonstration | 5 times per hour | __ consecutive trials out of __ | by: (__ days) |
| | -with less than 5 verbal prompts | 6 consecutive times per hour | 20% of the time | by: (1 week) |
| | -with less than 3 verbal prompts | 2 times per day | 50% of the time | by: (3 weeks) |
| | -with 1 verbal prompt | 3 times per day | ___% of the time | by: (1 month) |
| | -with maximum assistance | 6 times per day | | by: (6 weeks) |
| | -with moderate assistance | 1 time per week | | by: (8 weeks) |
| | -with minimum assistance | 3 times per week | | by: (3 months) |
| | -with ___% assistance | 8 times per week | | by: (__ months) |
| | -in the therapy setting | 1 time per month | | |
| | -in the home setting | 3 times per month | | |
| | -independently | 6 times per month | | |
| | -correctly | | | |
| | -accurately | | | |

© SLACK Inc.

## Therapeutic Suggestions

1. Provide a class on skin care. Discuss different skin types, lotions, and sunscreens. Ask members how to protect skin from medications, side effects, and weather conditions; add suggestions not mentioned by the group.

2. Have a class session on skin facials. Assist group members in making their own facials from recipes and materials provided in class. Have all members give self a complete facial including a massage. Discuss relaxation benefits of performing a facial as a stress management activity.

3. Have a class session on foot care. Discuss what a callous, bunion, rash, athletes foot, etc., is and what materials can treat specific foot ailments versus what requires a doctor's attention. Discuss how to prevent foot problems and the importance of well-designed functional shoes.

4. Develop an eye care class for individuals who have vision difficulties. Discuss different ways to adapt home or work environment to assist in independent living. Discuss different options available to improve sight (leader dogs, eyeglasses, contacts).

5. Have all members demonstrate how to clean glasses and/or contact lenses. Discuss ways to prevent scratching, tearing, or other damage to lenses. Compare and contrast the advantages and disadvantages of contact lenses versus glasses, including cost and insurance coverage for each individual.

6. Discuss eyeglass selection according to individual facial features. Plan an outing with one or two individuals visiting several stores to try on different eyeglass styles and compare cost before selection.

7. Develop an insurance education class. Have all members recognize what health insurance is, and discuss medical insurance coverage. Compare and contrast different levels of insurance coverage and where to call specific companies to ask health-related questions. Have group practice filling out insurance claim forms.

8. Have members practice calling physicians' offices to leave messages or make appointments. Discuss importance of writing down the date, time, and location of the appointment and placing it on a calendar.

9. Discuss in a health class the difference between a sign and symptom. Give group members signs and symptoms, have them guess the problem/ailment. Reverse and provide the problem/ailment, have group give signs and symptoms.

10. In health education class, discuss what a physical examination consists of and why one must be completed at least yearly. Practice filling out sample forms required by physicians' offices before an examination is conducted.

11. Discuss how to tell the difference between healthy and unhealthy teeth. Have each group member report one way to prevent cavities. Write down prevention ideas on blackboard or large sheet of paper; discuss how many of these members include in their daily routines.

12. Invite a dental hygienist to speak in health education class. Identify signs and symptoms of tooth problems and preventative techniques. Include a demonstration on how to brush teeth, floss correctly, and clean dentures. Provide a brief overview of how teeth cleaning is completed during office visits and the importance of regular check-ups.

13. Have group members practice brushing and flossing teeth in front of a mirror. Have members practice gargling with mouthwash. Discuss why brushing after every meal and flossing once daily is important.

14. Develop a medication class. Have a qualified health professional discuss the benefits of medication in controlling or reducing negative symptoms. Discuss side effects of medication and coping strategies.

15. In a role play situation, have group members practice verbalizing to a physician concerns regarding medication. Have members switch roles. Practice reporting medication side effects and negotiating problems and issues with physician.

16. Develop a family education/supportive others program. Involve group members and families in discussion of problems and difficulties that occur without medication and benefits associated with regular medication usage. Discuss how medication controls symptoms and side effects associated with usage.

17. Discuss with group members and families/supportive others the significance of maintaining the medical regime and the incorrect/negative attitude towards taking prescribed drugs as a sign of dependency and weak character. Encourage medication comparisons to other disabilities such as insulin to diabetics and nitroglycerine to heart patients. Reinforce belief of medication usage as a strength versus a weakness.

18. Develop a personal health class discussing the differences between male and female reproductive systems, including how conception occurs. Discuss different levels of birth control beginning with abstinence.

19. Discuss signs, symptoms, and how to prevent sexually transmitted diseases (STD) from occurring. Discuss Acquired Immune Deficiency Syndrome (AIDS); how it can and cannot be transmitted including methods of prevention.

20. Conduct a diet and exercise class. Discuss relationship between food, exercise and health. Examine all activities that provide exercise and have each member contract to increase their exercise level by _____ minutes per day. Reinforce goals met.

21. Provide a nutritional meal planning group. Have each member rotate for planning a complete, well-balanced, nutritional meal. Have member planning the menu shop for items and assign cooking duties to rest of participants.

22. Develop low impact aerobic and stretch and tone exercise classes. Place each participant based on evaluation and assessment of exercise level, physical capacity, and medical history. Have members lead certain components of exercise class. Emphasize good form and correct posture.

23. Develop a chart for members who volunteer to participate in a program to increase exercise levels. Place star or other reward by those who meet daily goal. Fine others $_____ per day for unmet goals.

24. Develop a stress management class. Discuss different ways of relaxing. Have members brainstorm additional techniques. Ask members to apply some of these ideas to stressful events in their own lives. Have members practice active and passive relaxation techniques, avoid guided imagery with persons suffering from serious mental illness.

25. Develop a body mechanics class; show members a skeleton or chart with anatomy of spine and supporting structures. Discuss relationship between all components in producing a healthy back.

26. Provide a demonstration on correct and incorrect sitting, standing, and sleeping postures. Demonstrate ways to perform daily living skills to prevent back injuries. Have all members practice correct lifting techniques and complete 30 minutes of back exercises.

# Chapter 14

# Life Safety

The purpose of this chapter is to provide an overview of skills required for the area of life safety. In order for an individual to live independently, there are skills that need to be addressed to prevent emergency situations. A variety of life skills is listed such as emergency assistance, home safety, and first aid. The category of home safety is further divided into areas of electrical/gas, fire, and poisons. The category of first aid is divided into cuts, burns, eye/nose injuries, seizures, temperature extremes, rescue breathing, choking, and CPR.

*Table 14-1*

| Life Safety | | | Objective | |
|---|---|---|---|---|
| **Behavioral Task** | **Condition of Performance** | **Frequency or Duration** | **Criteria for Moving to the Next Level of Performance** | **Time Frame** |
| **Emergency Assistance.**<br>The client will: | -with maximum physical guidance | | | |
| | -with moderate physical guidance | 1 time per minute | 1 out of 3 times | by: (1 hour) |
| Verbalize difference in policemen, firemen, and emergency medical services. | -with minimal physical guidance | 3 times per minute | 3 out of 6 times | by: (6 hours) |
| Verbalize how to contact each emergency service. | -with ___% physical guidance | 5 times per minute | __ out of __ times | by: (__ hours) |
| | -with tactile cues | 1 time per hour | 4 consecutive trials out of 8 | by: (1 day) |
| Locate in phone book emergency number closest to home environment. | -with a demonstration | 3 times per hour | 12 consecutive trials out of 15 | by: (3 days) |
| Verbalize when to call for emergency assistance. | -with less than 3 verbal prompts | 5 times per hour | __ consecutive trials out of __ | by: (__ days) |
| | -with 1 verbal prompt | 6 consecutive times per hour | 20% of the time | by: (1 week) |
| Post emergency numbers and address of residence by phone. | -with maximum assistance | 2 times per day | 50% of the time | by: (3 weeks) |
| Dial emergency number. | -with moderate assistance | 3 times per day | ___% of the time | by: (1 month) |
| Dial operator for assistance. | -with minimum assistance | 6 times per day | | by: (6 weeks) |
| Verbalize required steps of emergency assistance. | -with ___% assistance | 1 time per week | | by: (8 weeks) |
| | -in the therapy setting | 3 times per week | | by: (3 months) |
| Give accurate location of place and person when calling for emergency assistance. | -in a public setting | 8 times per week | | by: (__ months) |
| Describe injury and what happened to emergency service operator. | -in a community setting | 1 time per month | | |
| | -independently | 3 times per month | | |
| Hang up phone after emergency service operator. | -safely | 6 times per month | | |
| Remain calm when contacting emergency assistance. | -correctly | | | |

*Table 14-1 (Continued)*

| Life Safety | | | **Objective** | |
|---|---|---|---|---|
| **Behavioral Task** | **Condition of Performance** | **Frequency or Duration** | **Criteria for Moving to the Next Level of Performance** | **Time Frame** |
| Demonstrate required steps of providing emergency assistance. | -with maximum physical guidance | 1 time per minute | 1 out of 3 times | by: (1 hour) |
| | -with moderate physical guidance | 3 times per minute | 3 out of 6 times | by: (6 hours) |
| **Electrical/Gas.** The client will: | -with minimal physical guidance | 5 times per minute | __ out of __ times | by: (__ hours) |
| Point out objects that use electricity. | -with ___% physical guidance | 1 time per hour | 4 consecutive trials out of 8 | by: (1 day) |
| Point out electrical parts/components. | -with tactile cues | 3 times per hour | 12 consecutive trials out of 15 | by: (3 days) |
| Verbalize dangers of electricity. | -with a demonstration | 5 times per hour | __ consecutive trials out of __ | by: (__ days) |
| Dry hands before using electrical appliance. | -with less than 3 verbal prompts | 6 consecutive times per hour | 20% of the time | by: (1 week) |
| Place electrical appliances away from water. | -with 1 verbal prompt | 2 times per day | 50% of the time | by: (3 weeks) |
| Turn off electrical appliances when finished. | -with maximum assistance | 3 times per day | ___% of the time | by: (1 month) |
| Plug in electrical appliance correctly. | -with moderate assistance | 6 times per day | | by: (6 weeks) |
| Unplug electrical appliance. | -with minimum assistance | 1 time per week | | by: (8 weeks) |
| Recognize electrical appliance not working properly. | -with ___% assistance | 3 times per week | | by: (3 months) |
| Use electrical appliances. | -in the therapy setting | 8 times per week | | by: (__ months) |
| Follow rules of electrical safety. | -in a public setting | 1 time per month | | |
| Teach electrical safety skills to others. | -in a community setting | 3 times per month | | |
| Point out objects that use gas. | -independently | 6 times per month | | |
| Verbalize dangers of gas. | -safely | | | |
| Verbalize safety procedures when smelling gas. | -correctly | | | |

*Table 14-1 (Continued)*

| Life Safety | | Objective | | |
|---|---|---|---|---|
| **Behavioral Task** | **Condition of Performance** | **Frequency or Duration** | **Criteria for Moving to the Next Level of Performance** | **Time Frame** |
| Recognize smell of gas. | -with maximum physical guidance | 1 time per minute | 1 out of 3 times | by: (1 hour) |
| Know where to shut off gas flow. | -with moderate physical guidance | 3 times per minute | 3 out of 6 times | by: (6 hours) |
| Practice shutting off gas control. | -with minimal physical guidance | 5 times per minute | __ out of __ times | by: (__ hours) |
| Call power company to report gas smells. | -with ___% physical guidance | 1 time per hour | 4 consecutive trials out of 8 | by: (1 day) |
| Open windows to ventilate area. | -with tactile cues | 3 times per hour | 12 consecutive trials out of 15 | by: (3 days) |
| **Fire Safety.** The client will: | -with a demonstration | 5 times per hour | __ consecutive trials out of __ | by: (__ days) |
| Verbalize causes of home fires. | -with less than 3 verbal prompts | 6 consecutive times per hour | 20% of the time | by: (1 week) |
| Identify ways to prevent home fires. | -with 1 verbal prompt | 2 times per day | 50% of the time | by: (3 weeks) |
| Verbalize how to use a fire extinguisher. | -with maximum assistance | 3 times per day | ___% of the time | by: (1 month) |
| Operate a fire extinguisher. | -with moderate assistance | 6 times per day | | by: (6 weeks) |
| Recognize differences in fire extinguishers. | -with minimum assistance | 1 time per week | | by: (8 weeks) |
| Use correct extinguisher to stop fire. | -with ___% assistance | 3 times per week | | by: (3 months) |
| Verbalize how to put out an electrical, oil, or grease fire. | -in the therapy setting | 8 times per week | | by: (__ months) |
| Verbalize how to prevent home fires. | -in a public setting | 1 time per month | | |
| | -in a community setting | 3 times per month | | |
| **Poisons.** The client will: | -independently | 6 times per month | | |
| Define what a poison is. | -safely | | | |
| Recognize poisonous substances. | -correctly | | | |

*Table 14-1 (Continued)*

| Life Safety | Objective | | | |
|---|---|---|---|---|
| **Behavioral Task** | **Condition of Performance** | **Frequency or Duration** | **Criteria for Moving to the Next Level of Performance** | **Time Frame** |
| Recognize poisonous labels. | -with maximum physical guidance | 1 time per minute | 1 out of 3 times | by: (1 hour) |
| Identify poisonous substances in house. | -with moderate physical guidance | 3 times per minute | 3 out of 6 times | by: (6 hours) |
| Store poisonous substances in safe area. | -with minimal physical guidance | 5 times per minute | __ out of __ times | by: (__ hours) |
| Use poisonous substances only when necessary. | -with ___% physical guidance | 1 time per hour | 4 consecutive trials out of 8 | by: (1 day) |
| | -with tactile cues | 3 times per hour | 12 consecutive trials out of 15 | by: (3 days) |
| Recognize signs of a poisoning (nausea, vomiting, unconsciousness). | -with a demonstration | 5 times per hour | __ consecutive trials out of __ | by: (__ days) |
| Call Poison Control Center/Emergency Medical Services for immediate assistance if a poisoning occurs. | -with less than 3 verbal prompts | 6 consecutive times per hour | 20% of the time | by: (1 week) |
| | -with 1 verbal prompt | 2 times per day | 50% of the time | by: (3 weeks) |
| Verbalize causes of poison (plants, medicines, cleaning agents). | -with maximum assistance | 3 times per day | ___% of the time | by: (1 month) |
| | -with moderate assistance | 6 times per day | | by: (6 weeks) |
| Teach poison prevention skills to others. | -with minimum assistance | 1 time per week | | by: (8 weeks) |
| **Cuts.** The client will: | -with ___% assistance | 3 times per week | | by: (3 months) |
| Identify and verbalize cause of a cut. | -in the therapy setting | 8 times per week | | by: (__ months) |
| Verbalize how to prevent a cut from occurring. | -in a public setting | 1 time per month | | |
| Differentiate between major and minor cuts. | -in a community setting | 3 times per month | | |
| Verbalize what an infection is and signs of it. | -independently | 6 times per month | | |
| Report how to prevent an infection. | -safely | | | |
| | -correctly | | | |

© SLACK Inc.

*Table 14-1 (Continued)*

| Life Safety | | | **Objective** | |
|---|---|---|---|---|
| **Behavioral Task** | **Condition of Performance** | **Frequency or Duration** | **Criteria for Moving to the Next Level of Performance** | **Time Frame** |
| Demonstrate how to wash a cut with soap and water. | -with maximum physical guidance | 1 time per minute | 1 out of 3 times | by: (1 hour) |
| | -with moderate physical guidance | 3 times per minute | 3 out of 6 times | by: (6 hours) |
| Cover minor cut with band aid. | -with minimal physical guidance | 5 times per minute | __ out of __ times | by: (__ hours) |
| Verbalize why pressure is applied to a cut. | -with ___% physical guidance | 1 time per hour | 4 consecutive trials out of 8 | by: (1 day) |
| Verbalize steps to take when major cut occurs. | -with tactile cues | 3 times per hour | 12 consecutive trials out of 15 | by: (3 days) |
| **Burns.** The client will: | -with a demonstration | 5 times per hour | __ consecutive trials out of __ | by: (__ days) |
| Identify burn. | -with less than 3 verbal prompts | 6 consecutive times per hour | 20% of the time | by: (1 week) |
| Report how burns are classified. | -with 1 verbal prompt | 2 times per day | 50% of the time | by: (3 weeks) |
| Distinguish between first, second, and third degree burns. | -with maximum assistance | 3 times per day | ___% of the time | by: (1 month) |
| | -with moderate assistance | 6 times per day | | by: (6 weeks) |
| Verbalize how to treat first degree burn (cool water). | -with minimum assistance | 1 time per week | | by: (8 weeks) |
| Verbalize how to treat second and third degree burns (dry bandages, hospital). | -with ___% assistance | 3 times per week | | by: (3 months) |
| | -in the therapy setting | 8 times per week | | by: (__ months) |
| Report all necessary steps to take when burn occurs. | -in a public setting | 1 time per month | | |
| **Eye/Nose Injuries.** The client will: | -in a community setting | 3 times per month | | |
| Identify cause of eye injuries. | -independently | 6 times per month | | |
| Verbalize how to prevent eye injuries. | -safely | | | |
| | -correctly | | | |

Table 14-1 (Continued)

| Life Safety | Objective | | | |
|---|---|---|---|---|
| **Behavioral Task** | **Condition of Performance** | **Frequency or Duration** | **Criteria for Moving to the Next Level of Performance** | **Time Frame** |
| Recognize signs and symptoms of eye injury. | -with maximum physical guidance | 1 time per minute | 1 out of 3 times | by: (1 hour) |
| Demonstrate how to bandage an eye injury. | -with moderate physical guidance | 3 times per minute | 3 out of 6 times | by: (6 hours) |
| Demonstrate how to wash/rinse injured eye. | -with minimal physical guidance | 5 times per minute | __ out of __ times | by: (__ hours) |
| Recognize when to go to hospital. | -with ___% physical guidance | 1 time per hour | 4 consecutive trials out of 8 | by: (1 day) |
| Identify causes of a nosebleed. | -with tactile cues | 3 times per hour | 12 consecutive trials out of 15 | by: (3 days) |
| Verbalize and demonstrate how to control a nosebleed. | -with a demonstration | 5 times per hour | __ consecutive trials out of __ | by: (__ days) |
| | -with less than 3 verbal prompts | 6 consecutive times per hour | 20% of the time | by: (1 week) |
| Verbalize when not to control a nosebleed (patient has back, neck, or head injury). | -with 1 verbal prompt | 2 times per day | 50% of the time | by: (3 weeks) |
| Verbalize all steps to take when eye injury or nosebleed occurs. | -with maximum assistance | 3 times per day | ___% of the time | by: (1 month) |
| | -with moderate assistance | 6 times per day | | by: (6 weeks) |
| **Fractures, Dislocations, Sprains, Strains.** The client will: | -with minimum assistance | 1 time per week | | by: (8 weeks) |
| | -with ___% assistance | 3 times per week | | by: (3 months) |
| Identify causes of fracture. | -in the therapy setting | 8 times per week | | by: (__ months) |
| Differentiate between open and closed fractures. | -in a public setting | 1 time per month | | |
| Identify signs and symptoms of a fracture (swelling, bruising, pain) and how to prevent one from occurring. | -in a community setting | 3 times per month | | |
| | -independently | 6 times per month | | |
| Define dislocation and how to prevent one from occurring. | -safely | | | |
| Identify signs, symptoms, and causes of dislocation. | -correctly | | | |

*Table 14-1 (Continued)*

| Life Safety | Objective | | | |
|---|---|---|---|---|
| **Behavioral Task** | **Condition of Performance** | **Frequency or Duration** | **Criteria for Moving to the Next Level of Performance** | **Time Frame** |
| Define and identify causes of a sprain (falls, sports injury) and how to prevent one from occurring. | -with maximum physical guidance | 1 time per minute | 1 out of 3 times | by: (1 hour) |
| | -with moderate physical guidance | 3 times per minute | 3 out of 6 times | by: (6 hours) |
| Distinguish between a sprain and strain. | -with minimal physical guidance | 5 times per minute | __ out of __ times | by: (__ hours) |
| Identify causes of strain (lifting improperly). | -with ___% physical guidance | 1 time per hour | 4 consecutive trials out of 8 | by: (1 day) |
| Verbalize purpose of splinting and watch how to make a splint. | -with tactile cues | 3 times per hour | 12 consecutive trials out of 15 | by: (3 days) |
| | -with a demonstration | 5 times per hour | __ consecutive trials out of __ | by: (__ days) |
| Make a splint for a leg fracture. | -with less than 3 verbal prompts | 6 consecutive times per hour | 20% of the time | by: (1 week) |
| Differentiate when and when not to splint. | -with 1 verbal prompt | 2 times per day | 50% of the time | by: (3 weeks) |
| Verbalize and practice all steps to follow when fracture, dislocation, sprain, or strain occurs. | -with maximum assistance | 3 times per day | ___% of the time | by: (1 month) |
| **Seizures.** The client will: | -with moderate assistance | 6 times per day | | by: (6 weeks) |
| Identify causes of a seizure (shock, fever, head injury). | -with minimum assistance | 1 time per week | | by: (8 weeks) |
| | -with ___% assistance | 3 times per week | | by: (3 months) |
| Recognize signs and symptoms of a seizure. | -in the therapy setting | 8 times per week | | by: (__ months) |
| Identify when to call for assistance when a seizure occurs. | -in a public setting | 1 time per month | | |
| Identify when not to call for assistance. | -in a community setting | 3 times per month | | |
| Remove objects near person having seizure for safety. | -independently | 6 times per month | | |
| | -safely | | | |
| Verbalize and practice rolling victim on side if vomiting occurs. | -correctly | | | |

*Table 14-1 (Continued)*

| Life Safety | Objective | | | |
|---|---|---|---|---|
| **Behavioral Task** | **Condition of Performance** | **Frequency or Duration** | **Criteria for Moving to the Next Level of Performance** | **Time Frame** |
| Verbalize need to stay with victim until full consciousness occurs. | -with maximum physical guidance | 1 time per minute | 1 out of 3 times | by: (1 hour) |
| | -with moderate physical guidance | 3 times per minute | 3 out of 6 times | by: (6 hours) |
| Report to significant other when seizure occurs. | -with minimal physical guidance | 5 times per minute | __ out of __ times | by: (__ hours) |
| **Temperature Extremes.** | -with ___% physical guidance | 1 time per hour | 4 consecutive trials out of 8 | by: (1 day) |
| The client will: | -with tactile cues | 3 times per hour | 12 consecutive trials out of 15 | by: (3 days) |
| Identify causes of heat stroke. | -with a demonstration | 5 times per hour | __ consecutive trials out of __ | by: (__ days) |
| Verbalize signs and symptoms of heat stroke (small pupils, red skin). | -with less than 3 verbal prompts | 6 consecutive times per hour | 20% of the time | by: (1 week) |
| Identify heat exhaustion. | -with 1 verbal prompt | 2 times per day | 50% of the time | by: (3 weeks) |
| Differentiate between heat stroke and heat exhaustion. | -with maximum assistance | 3 times per day | ___% of the time | by: (1 month) |
| | -with moderate assistance | 6 times per day | | by: (6 weeks) |
| Verbalize signs and symptoms of heat exhaustion. | -with minimum assistance | 1 time per week | | by: (8 weeks) |
| Identify heat cramps. | -with ___% assistance | 3 times per week | | by: (3 months) |
| Verbalize signs and symptoms of heat cramps. | -in the therapy setting | 8 times per week | | by: (__ months) |
| Identify hypothermia. | -in a public setting | 1 time per month | | |
| Verbalize signs and symptoms of hypothermia. | -in a community setting | 3 times per month | | |
| Recognize signs of frost bite. | -independently | 6 times per month | | |
| Verbalize steps needed to follow when heat stroke, heat exhaustion, heat cramps, frost bite, and hypothermia occur. | -safely | | | |
| | -correctly | | | |

*Table 14-1 (Continued)*

| *Life Safety* | **Objective** | | | |
|---|---|---|---|---|
| **Behavioral Task** | **Condition of Performance** | **Frequency or Duration** | **Criteria for Moving to the Next Level of Performance** | **Time Frame** |
| Demonstrate steps required to follow when extreme temperature injury occurs. | -with maximum physical guidance | 1 time per minute | 1 out of 3 times | by: (1 hour) |
| | -with moderate physical guidance | 3 times per minute | 3 out of 6 times | by: (6 hours) |
| **Rescue Breathing.** The client will: | -with minimal physical guidance | 5 times per minute | __ out of __ times | by: (__ hours) |
| Verbalize definition of rescue breathing/artificial respiration. | -with ___% physical guidance | 1 time per hour | 4 consecutive trials out of 8 | by: (1 day) |
| Identify causes of breathing emergencies (poisons, drowning, drugs, burns, shock). | -with tactile cues | 3 times per hour | 12 consecutive trials out of 15 | by: (3 days) |
| | -with a demonstration | 5 times per hour | __ consecutive trials out of __ | by: (__ days) |
| Verbalize how to check for unresponsiveness. | -with less than 3 verbal prompts | 6 consecutive times per hour | 20% of the time | by: (1 week) |
| Verbalize how to position unconscious victim. | -with 1 verbal prompt | 2 times per day | 50% of the time | by: (3 weeks) |
| Demonstrate how to position unconscious victim. | -with maximum assistance | 3 times per day | ___% of the time | by: (1 month) |
| Demonstrate how to open the airway. | -with moderate assistance | 6 times per day | | by: (6 weeks) |
| Demonstrate how to look, listen, and feel for breathing. | -with minimum assistance | 1 time per week | | by: (8 weeks) |
| Give two breaths to unconscious victim. | -with ___% assistance | 3 times per week | | by: (3 months) |
| Identify where to check carotid pulse. | -in the therapy setting | 8 times per week | | by: (__ months) |
| Demonstrate how to check carotid pulse. | -in a public setting | 1 time per month | | |
| Verbalize when not to give rescue breathing. | -in a community setting | 3 times per month | | |
| Verbalize when to call emergency medical service for assistance. | -independently | 6 times per month | | |
| | -safely | | | |
| | -correctly | | | |

*Table 14-1 (Continued)*

| Life Safety | Objective | | | |
|---|---|---|---|---|
| **Behavioral Task** | **Condition of Performance** | **Frequency or Duration** | **Criteria for Moving to the Next Level of Performance** | **Time Frame** |
| **Choking.** The client will: | | | | |
| Verbalize definition of choking. | -with maximum physical guidance | 1 time per minute | 1 out of 3 times | by: (1 hour) |
| Identify common causes of choking. | -with moderate physical guidance | 3 times per minute | 3 out of 6 times | by: (6 hours) |
| Report signs and symptoms of choking. | -with minimal physical guidance | 5 times per minute | __ out of __ times | by: (__ hours) |
| Differentiate between partial and complete airway obstruction. | -with ___% physical guidance | 1 time per hour | 4 consecutive trials out of 8 | by: (1 day) |
| | -with tactile cues | 3 times per hour | 12 consecutive trials out of 15 | by: (3 days) |
| Verbalize the universal distress signal for choking. | -with a demonstration | 5 times per hour | __ consecutive trials out of __ | by: (__ days) |
| Identify and demonstrate first aid steps in conscious victim. | -with less than 3 verbal prompts | 6 consecutive times per hour | 20% of the time | by: (1 week) |
| | -with 1 verbal prompt | 2 times per day | 50% of the time | by: (3 weeks) |
| Perform abdominal thrust technique. | -with maximum assistance | 3 times per day | ___% of the time | by: (1 month) |
| Demonstrate first aid steps in unconscious victim. | -with moderate assistance | 6 times per day | | by: (6 weeks) |
| Perform finger sweep. | -with minimum assistance | 1 time per week | | by: (8 weeks) |
| Perform chest thrusts. | -with ___% assistance | 3 times per week | | by: (3 months) |
| Identify how to help self if alone and choking. | -in a public setting | 8 times per week | | by: (__ months) |
| **CPR.** The client will: | -in a community setting | 1 time per month | | |
| Verbalize definition of heart attack. | -independently | 3 times per month | | |
| Verbalize definition of cardiac arrest. | -safely | 6 times per month | | |
| Report signs and symptoms of heart attack (sweating, nausea). | -correctly | | | |

*Table 14-1 (Continued)*

| Life Safety | | Objective | | |
|---|---|---|---|---|
| **Behavioral Task** | **Condition of Performance** | **Frequency or Duration** | **Criteria for Moving to the Next Level of Performance** | **Time Frame** |
| Verbalize importance of phoning emergency medical services for assistance. | -with maximum physical guidance | 1 time per minute | 1 out of 3 times | by: (1 hour) |
| Verbalize what CPR stands for. | -with moderate physical guidance | 3 times per minute | 3 out of 6 times | by: (6 hours) |
| Demonstrate technique of one person CPR. | -with minimal physical guidance | 5 times per minute | __ out of __ times | by: (__ hours) |
| Demonstrate technique of two person CPR. | -with ___% physical guidance | 1 time per hour | 4 consecutive trials out of 8 | by: (1 day) |
| Verbalize risk factors of heart disease. | -with tactile cues | 3 times per hour | 12 consecutive trials out of 15 | by: (3 days) |
| Differentiate between changeable and unchangeable risk factors for heart disease. | -with a demonstration | 5 times per hour | __ consecutive trials out of __ | by: (__ days) |
| | -with less than 3 verbal prompts | 6 consecutive times per hour | 20% of the time | by: (1 week) |
| Verbalize how to prevent heart disease. | -with 1 verbal prompt | 2 times per day | 50% of the time | by: (3 weeks) |
| Verbalize how to change own lifestyle to prevent heart disease. | -with maximum assistance | 3 times per day | ___% of the time | by: (1 month) |
| Change one high-risk behavior to prevent heart disease. | -with moderate assistance | 6 times per day | | by: (6 weeks) |
| | -with minimum assistance | 1 time per week | | by: (8 weeks) |
| Attend and complete American Red Cross first aid class and receive certificate. | -with ___% assistance | 3 times per week | | by: (3 months) |
| | -in the therapy setting | 8 times per week | | by: (__ months) |
| Attend and complete American Red Cross CPR class and receive certificate. | -in a public setting | 1 time per month | | |
| Attend American Red Cross instructors class. | -in a community setting | 3 times per month | | |
| Receive an American Red Cross teacher's certificate. | -independently | 6 times per month | | |
| | -safely | | | |
| | -correctly | | | |

## Therapeutic Suggestions

1. Place phone books in the group setting, have group look for emergency service numbers (police, rescue, fire) nearest to their homes. Have them write numbers on paper and discuss where to post in home.

2. Place two phones in room; have each group member practice calling emergency service numbers for assistance. Practice giving all the necessary details of simulated accident, hang up after emergency operator.

3. Write down a variety of accident scenarios. Have each member pick one out of a hat and discuss steps to take for emergency assistance. Have group provide feedback on accuracy of decisions.

4. Develop a fire and safety awareness day of the week. Have groups develop lists of causes of home fires. Make up signs to post in area of each cause of home fire and how to prevent it. Have all involved practice using fire extinguisher. Call area fire department for speaker or demonstration.

5. Take group to local poison control center. Ask for short presentation on poison prevention and awareness. Collect poison control information to share with family and friends.

6. Develop a poison awareness class. Ask each member to write down poisonous substances they have at home. List all on overhead projector or chalkboard; add others that are missing. Discuss where/how to store poisons, what to do if poisoning occurs.

7. Have individuals identify why it is important to know first aid. Have each member develop a first aid kit to use in the home.

8. Make up a first aid kit. Take out one or two items, ask group what is missing. Repeat activity; give out prizes to fill first aid kits.

9. Identify all items in First Aid kit and for what each item is used.

10. Have group brainstorm when and where accidents occur. Name places to keep a first aid kit for emergencies.

11. Write down a variety of scenarios on individuals who have cut themselves. Have each member pick scenario out of hat and discuss how accident could be prevented and what should be done immediately to stop bleeding. If unsure, members can ask one person in group for assistance.

12. Have members of group make a large picture collage to fit one wall. Have the collage made up of a situation that may cause burn injury to occur. After each situation have picture on how to prevent injury from occurring. Use collage as an exhibit on safety awareness week.

13. Have group members listen to difference of first, second, and third degree burns and how to treat them. Have members role play an accident with one person applying first aid procedure depending on description of burn and depth of injury. Have members switch roles from victim to rescuer.

14. Have group talk of experiences where they or a family member have fractured, dislocated, sprained, or strained a body part. Discuss if accident could have been prevented and how.

15. Mix up words strain, sprain, fracture, and dislocation. Have members pick out word, define it to group, and develop a situation which may cause this injury to occur.

16. Educate members on purposes of splinting and when to use in emergency situations. Have each member practice applying arm splint and leg splint on partner.

17. Discuss different types of seizures and what signs and symptoms look like. Identify precautions taken when individual has a seizure and who to call for assistance.

18. Give group members list of signs and symptoms of heat stroke, heat exhaustion, heat cramps, hypothermia, and frost bite. Have each member verbalize two situations which could cause these signs and symptoms to occur. Place all situations developed into hat; have each subgroup of two members pick situation and role play first aid steps needed for injury.

19. Have group members describe behaviors of person who appears unconscious. Discuss different causes of unconsciousness and how to check for breathing. Have each member in group check his own carotid pulse and then check person to the right.

20. Give members definition of choking and ask each person to give two common causes of why choking occurs. Brainstorm how to prevent choking accidents from happening. Discuss Heimlich maneuver and how to perform it on self and others.

21. Ask members to guess the universal sign for choking and what steps to take if they see a person in this situation. Discuss when not to help or provide assistance if person is choking.

22. Develop a health awareness group and have members draw signs and pictures on how to prevent heart disease. Develop pictures that compare and contrast healthy and unhealthy lifestyles. Have each member discuss ways to change own lifestyle and how others may be helpful and supportive.

23. Have members attend an American Red Cross class on First Aid and Cardio-Pulmonary Resuscitation and receive certificates for successful completion.

24. Have qualified and interested group members become trained as American Red Cross instructors, training peers in First Aid and CPR.

25. Practice fire drills at apartments, wards, and group homes.

26. Tour a fire department.

# Chapter 15

# Work-Related Skills

The purpose of this chapter is to provide a variety of work-related objectives to assist in developing and increasing vocational skills required for independent living. The objectives developed in this chapter address the areas of prevocational and vocational activities including work performance, vocational exploration, job acquisition, and retirement planning.

Persons who receive mental health services must be provided with the opportunity to actively participate in work programming. The literature clearly demonstrates that the opportunity to work has been correlated to a decrease in psychopathological symptoms (Jacobs, Karadashian, Kreinbring, Ponder & Simpson, 1984), as well as a decrease in psychiatric readmission rates (Franklin, Kittredge & Thrasher, 1975; Rubin & Roessler, 1978). Because of these important benefits, all health care providers must provide a concerted effort to develop and increase vocational programs available in community-based settings. Not all individuals are able to work independently and may require programs that are designed for their specific functional levels. A variety of levels exist to facilitate independent work behaviors such as sheltered employment, enclaves, mobile work crews, and supported employment programs. An individual may not need to progress through all levels of employment. A functional assessment to determine specific skill levels is necessary to provide a vocational program based on individual needs. Once an individual is assessed regarding vocational strengths, limitations, and performance level, an independent living skills program can be initiated.

*Table 15-1*

| Work-Related Skills | | Objective | | |
|---|---|---|---|---|
| **Behavioral Task** | **Condition of Performance** | **Frequency or Duration** | **Criteria for Moving to the Next Level of Performance** | **Time Frame** |
| **Work.** The client will: | | | | |
| Recognize work site and work station. | -with maximum physical guidance | 1 time per minute | 1 out of 3 times | by: (1 hour) |
| Walk to work with escort. | -with moderate physical guidance | 3 times per minute | 3 out of 6 times | by: (6 hours) |
| Walk to work without escort. | -with minimal physical guidance | 5 times per minute | __ out of __ times | by: (__ hours) |
| Assist new employee in finding work site. | -with ___% physical guidance | 1 time per hour | 4 consecutive trials out of 8 | by: (1 day) |
| Recognize time clock and card. | -with tactile cues | 3 times per hour | 12 consecutive trials out of 15 | by: (3 days) |
| Fill out time card legibly. | -with a demonstration | 5 times per hour | __ consecutive trials out of __ | by: (__ days) |
| Arrive to work less than 7 minutes late. | -with less than 3 verbal prompts | 6 consecutive times per hour | 20% of the time | by: (1 week) |
| Arrive to work less than 5 minutes late. | -with 1 verbal prompt | 2 times per day | 50% of the time | by: (3 weeks) |
| Arrive to work on time. | -with maximum assistance | 3 times per day | ___% of the time | by: (1 month) |
| Set up work station. | -with moderate assistance | 6 times per day | | by: (6 weeks) |
| Recognize work parts missing and verbally request work parts when needed. | -with minimum assistance | 1 time per week | | by: (8 weeks) |
| Recognize all parts of an assembled product. | -with ___% assistance | 3 times per week | | by: (3 months) |
| Produce a 2-3 part assembled product. | -with accuracy | 8 times per week | | by: (__ months) |
| Produce an 8-10 part assembled product. | -in the therapy setting | 1 time per month | | |
| Count 20 items of a product. | -in a vocational setting | 3 times per month | | |
| Collate 2 or more items. | -independently | 6 times per month | | |
| | -safely | | | |
| | -correctly | | | |

© SLACK Inc.

*Table 15-1 (Continued)*

| Work-Related Skills | Objective | | | |
|---|---|---|---|---|
| **Behavioral Task** | **Condition of Performance** | **Frequency or Duration** | **Criteria for Moving to the Next Level of Performance** | **Time Frame** |
| Collate a complete package without errors. | -with maximum physical guidance | 1 time per minute | 1 out of 3 times | by: (1 hour) |
| Staple 2-6 items. | -with moderate physical guidance | 3 times per minute | 3 out of 6 times | by: (6 hours) |
| Staple more than 10 items. | -with minimal physical guidance | 5 times per minute | __ out of __ times | by: (__ hours) |
| Punch 3 holes in __ sheets of paper. | -with ___% physical guidance | 1 time per hour | 4 consecutive trials out of 8 | by: (1 day) |
| Package more than 1-15 items. | -with tactile cues | 3 times per hour | 12 consecutive trials out of 15 | by: (3 days) |
| Count and collate 8 items. | -with a demonstration | 5 times per hour | __ consecutive trials out of __ | by: (__ days) |
| Collate, staple, and package 10 items. | -with less than 3 verbal prompts | 6 consecutive times per hour | 20% of the time | by: (1 week) |
| Count, collate, staple, and package an assembled product. | -with 1 verbal prompt | 2 times per day | 50% of the time | by: (3 weeks) |
| | -with maximum assistance | 3 times per day | ___% of the time | by: (1 month) |
| Wrap packages for delivery. | -with moderate assistance | 6 times per day | | by: (6 weeks) |
| Assist in delivering packages to designated area. | -with minimum assistance | 1 time per week | | by: (8 weeks) |
| Deliver __ package(s) to designated area. | -with ___% assistance | 3 times per week | | by: (3 months) |
| Escort other employees in delivering packages. | -with accuracy | 8 times per week | | by: (__ months) |
| | -in the therapy setting | 1 time per month | | |
| Recognize and use a screwdriver. | -in a vocational setting | 3 times per month | | |
| Recognize and use a wrench. | -independently | 6 times per month | | |
| Recognize and use a hammer. | -safely | | | |
| Recognize and use a hand saw. | -correctly | | | |

© SLACK Inc.

*Table 15-1 (Continued)*

| Work-Related Skills | | Objective | | |
|---|---|---|---|---|
| **Behavioral Task** | **Condition of Performance** | **Frequency or Duration** | **Criteria for Moving to the Next Level of Performance** | **Time Frame** |
| Recognize and use all non-powered hand tools. | -with maximum physical guidance | 1 time per minute | 1 out of 3 times | by: (1 hour) |
| Recognize power equipment. | -with moderate physical guidance | 3 times per minute | 3 out of 6 times | by: (6 hours) |
| Recognize all parts of desired power equipment. | -with minimal physical guidance | 5 times per minute | __ out of __ times | by: (__ hours) |
| | -with ___% physical guidance | 1 time per hour | 4 consecutive trials out of 8 | by: (1 day) |
| Recognize safety procedures for operating power equipment. | -with tactile cues | 3 times per hour | 12 consecutive trials out of 15 | by: (3 days) |
| Recognize and use safety procedures for operating power equipment. | -with a demonstration | 5 times per hour | __ consecutive trials out of __ | by: (__ days) |
| Operate rivet machine. | -with less than 3 verbal prompts | 6 consecutive times per hour | 20% of the time | by: (1 week) |
| Rivet all parts needed to complete product. | -with 1 verbal prompt | 2 times per day | 50% of the time | by: (3 weeks) |
| Recognize and operate a drill press. | -with maximum assistance | 3 times per day | ___% of the time | by: (1 month) |
| Drill all parts needed to complete product. | -with moderate assistance | 6 times per day | | by: (6 weeks) |
| Recognize and operate a band saw. | -with minimum assistance | 1 time per week | | by: (8 weeks) |
| Recognize and operate table saw. | -with ___% assistance | 3 times per week | | by: (3 months) |
| Rivet and drill desired piece of wood. | -with accuracy | 8 times per week | | by: (__ months) |
| Rivet, drill, and operate table saw. | -in the therapy setting | 1 time per month | | |
| Complete finished product using all power equipment. | -in a vocational setting | 3 times per month | | |
| | -independently | 6 times per month | | |
| Clean equipment used. | -safely | | | |
| Put equipment in desired location. | -correctly | | | |

*Table 15-1 (Continued)*

| Work-Related Skills | Objective | | | |
|---|---|---|---|---|
| **Behavioral Task** | **Condition of Performance** | **Frequency or Duration** | **Criteria for Moving to the Next Level of Performance** | **Time Frame** |
| Replace work parts. | -with maximum physical guidance | 1 time per minute | 1 out of 3 times | by: (1 hour) |
| Stock, sweep, dust, and mop work station. | -with moderate physical guidance | 3 times per minute | 3 out of 6 times | by: (6 hours) |
| Maintain clean work station. | -with minimal physical guidance | 5 times per minute | __ out of __ times | by: (__ hours) |
| Attend __ out of __ scheduled work days. | -with ___% physical guidance | 1 time per hour | 4 consecutive trials out of 8 | by: (1 day) |
| Attend all scheduled work days. | -with tactile cues | 3 times per hour | 12 consecutive trials out of 15 | by: (3 days) |
| Show up to work when scheduled. | -with a demonstration | 5 times per hour | __ consecutive trials out of __ | by: (__ days) |
| Notify supervisor when late. | -with less than 3 verbal prompts | 6 consecutive times per hour | 20% of the time | by: (1 week) |
| When ill notify supervisor before scheduled work time. | -with 1 verbal prompt | 2 times per day | 50% of the time | by: (3 weeks) |
| | -with maximum assistance | 3 times per day | ___% of the time | by: (1 month) |
| Work overtime when needed. | -with moderate assistance | 6 times per day | | by: (6 weeks) |
| Take breaks when assigned. | -with minimum assistance | 1 time per week | | by: (8 weeks) |
| Complete task with verbal instructions. | -with ___% assistance | 3 times per week | | by: (3 months) |
| Complete task with written instructions. | -with accuracy | 8 times per week | | by: (__ months) |
| Complete task with written diagrams. | -in the therapy setting | 1 time per month | | |
| Request assistance when unable to complete task. | -in a vocational setting | 3 times per month | | |
| Contact supervisor when mistake is made. | -independently | 6 times per month | | |
| Follow male and female supervisors' instructions. | -safely | | | |
| | -correctly | | | |

*Table 15-1 (Continued)*

| Work-Related Skills | Objective | | | |
|---|---|---|---|---|
| **Behavioral Task** | **Condition of Performance** | **Frequency or Duration** | **Criteria for Moving to the Next Level of Performance** | **Time Frame** |
| Accept directions, suggestions, and feedback from supervisor. | -with maximum physical guidance | 1 time per minute | 1 out of 3 times | by: (1 hour) |
| | -with moderate physical guidance | 3 times per minute | 3 out of 6 times | by: (6 hours) |
| Express work concerns without anger or yelling. | -with minimal physical guidance | 5 times per minute | __ out of __ times | by: (__ hours) |
| Follow developed job aid. | -with ___% physical guidance | 1 time per hour | 4 consecutive trials out of 8 | by: (1 day) |
| Complete task assigned. | -with tactile cues | 3 times per hour | 12 consecutive trials out of 15 | by: (3 days) |
| Assist co-workers in completing tasks. | -with a demonstration | 5 times per hour | __ consecutive trials out of __ | by: (__ days) |
| Interact with peers positively. | -with less than 3 verbal prompts | 6 consecutive times per hour | 20% of the time | by: (1 week) |
| Work well in group setting and alone. | -with 1 verbal prompt | 2 times per day | 50% of the time | by: (3 weeks) |
| Accept feedback from and provide feedback to co-workers. | -with maximum assistance | 3 times per day | ___% of the time | by: (1 month) |
| | -with moderate assistance | 6 times per day | | by: (6 weeks) |
| Lead co-workers to complete group task. | -with minimum assistance | 1 time per week | | by: (8 weeks) |
| Watch film on proper body mechanics. | -with ___% assistance | 3 times per week | | by: (3 months) |
| Recognize and verbalize principles of proper body mechanics. | -with accuracy | 8 times per week | | by: (__ months) |
| Identify poor back posture; bend correctly while working. | -in the therapy setting | 1 time per month | | |
| | -in a vocational setting | 3 times per month | | |
| Lift __ - __ pounds according to doctor's orders. | -independently | 6 times per month | | |
| Wear proper and comfortable work shoes. | -safely | | | |
| Attend job finding/employment skills classes. | -correctly | | | |

*Table 15-1  (Continued)*

| Work-Related Skills | Objective | | | |
| --- | --- | --- | --- | --- |
| **Behavioral Task** | **Condition of Performance** | **Frequency or Duration** | **Criteria for Moving to the Next Level of Performance** | **Time Frame** |
| Identify and verbalize vocational strengths and weaknesses. | -with maximum physical guidance | 1 time per minute | 1 out of 3 times | by: (1 hour) |
| | -with moderate physical guidance | 3 times per minute | 3 out of 6 times | by: (6 hours) |
| Listen to what employers expect from employees. | -with minimal physical guidance | 5 times per minute | __ out of __ times | by: (__ hours) |
| Verbalize employer expectations. | -with ___% physical guidance | 1 time per hour | 4 consecutive trials out of 8 | by: (1 day) |
| Listen to and verbalize effective methods of gathering job leads. | -with tactile cues | 3 times per hour | 12 consecutive trials out of 15 | by: (3 days) |
| | -with a demonstration | 5 times per hour | __ consecutive trials out of __ | by: (__ days) |
| Practice effective methods of gathering job leads. | -with less than 3 verbal prompts | 6 consecutive times per hour | 20% of the time | by: (1 week) |
| Use time effectively in gathering job leads. | -with 1 verbal prompt | 2 times per day | 50% of the time | by: (3 weeks) |
| Recognize and complete a job application. | -with maximum assistance | 3 times per day | ___% of the time | by: (1 month) |
| Pick up three blank job applications from area businesses. | -with moderate assistance | 6 times per day | | by: (6 weeks) |
| Deliver application to desired business. | -with minimum assistance | 1 time per week | | by: (8 weeks) |
| Call potential employer on telephone. | -with ___% assistance | 3 times per week | | by: (3 months) |
| Verbalize skills and abilities to potential employer. | -with accuracy | 8 times per week | | by: (__ months) |
| | -in the therapy setting | 1 time per month | | |
| Secure job interview with potential employer. | -in a vocational setting | 3 times per month | | |
| Watch tape on interviewing and verbalize principles on how to interview. | -independently | 6 times per month | | |
| | -safely | | | |
| Answer problem questions. | -correctly | | | |

*Table 15-1 (Continued)*

| Work Related Skills | Objective | | | |
|---|---|---|---|---|
| **Behavioral Task** | **Condition of Performance** | **Frequency or Duration** | **Criteria for Moving to the Next Level of Performance** | **Time Frame** |
| Recognize a functional and a chronological resume. | -with maximum physical guidance | 1 time per minute | 1 out of 3 times | by: (1 hour) |
| Recognize the difference between the two resumes. | -with moderate physical guidance | 3 times per minute | 3 out of 6 times | by: (6 hours) |
| | -with minimal physical guidance | 5 times per minute | __ out of __ times | by: (__ hours) |
| Prepare and complete a resume. | -with ___% physical guidance | 1 time per hour | 4 consecutive trials out of 8 | by: (1 day) |
| Deliver application to employer and secure interview time. | -with tactile cues | 3 times per hour | 12 consecutive trials out of 15 | by: (3 days) |
| Interview with employer and attain employment. | -with a demonstration | 5 times per hour | __ consecutive trials out of __ | by: (__ days) |
| | -with less than 3 verbal prompts | 6 consecutive times per hour | 20% of the time | by: (1 week) |
| Verbalize and be aware of principles of supported employment. | -with 1 verbal prompt | 2 times per day | 50% of the time | by: (3 weeks) |
| | -with maximum assistance | 3 times per day | ___% of the time | by: (1 month) |
| Recognize difference between enclave and work crew. | -with moderate assistance | 6 times per day | | by: (6 weeks) |
| Recognize difference between job coach and job trainer. | -with minimum assistance | 1 time per week | | by: (8 weeks) |
| Participate in supported employment setting. | -with ___% assistance | 3 times per week | | by: (3 months) |
| Work in job without supports. | -with accuracy | 8 times per week | | by: (__ months) |
| Attend retirement seminar. | -in the therapy setting | 1 time per month | | |
| Determine aptitudes, interests, and skills. | -in a vocational setting | 3 times per month | | |
| Identify vocational pursuits. | -independently | 6 times per month | | |
| Write a retirement plan. | -safely | | | |
| | -correctly | | | |

## Therapeutic Suggestions

1. Provide client with a simulated work environment to train on the use of power equipment. Do not plug in any of the machinery to assess safety skills. Have client verbalize how to operate band saw, table saw, rivet machine, and drill press.

2. Provide a videotape of maintaining and cleaning equipment. Then videotape client performing same duties.

3. Demonstrate to client how to set up and stock a work station. Have client identify supplies and parts missing in an unstocked work station.

4. Provide a chart with each worker's name on it. When worker is on time, place star by his or her name.

5. Institute a program with "worker of the month." Have work supervisors and peers vote together.

6. Give monthly certificates for workers with high levels of punctuality and dependability.

7. Give work instruction verbally, in writing, and on a videotaped program. Reinforce all appropriate work behaviors immediately after they have occurred.

8. Videotape examples of worker's response to supervision, showing correct and incorrect ways of addressing problems. Ask client which behavior will have a more positive outcome.

9. Assign workers of different functional levels to complete a task together. Role model team work concept and praise each client's behavior as it resembles team work and co-worker's behavior.

10. Have clients attend group on accepting and providing feedback to others. Have each member practice same example and immediately reinforce correct response.

11. Have client view a tape on proper body mechanics. Provide instructions and role modeling on proper lifting techniques. Ask clients to lift objects in the setting demonstrating correct and incorrect responses.

12. Have clients brainstorm where to find job leads in the community. Add ideas and suggestions, if necessary, emphasizing the method of networking and informal contacts.

13. Have clients practice community mobility techniques to get to a job.

14. Have clients go to community and ask area businesses for job applications. Have each client fill out an application. Go over applications individually, recommending improvements.

15. Have clients practice telephone calling. Set up two telephones designating one client to be the employer and the other client as employee. Reinforce appropriate conversation skills immediately following the desired behavior.

16. Show a videotape on clients involved in supported employment programs; have clients verbalize benefits involved in this model. Provide resources to clients on how to become involved in a supported employment program.

17. Assist client to ride bus to local rehabilitation office to apply for vocational assistance.

18. Have clients ride bus to the local employment security commission to register for employment opportunities.

19. Have a discussion group regarding references for employment. Explore advantages and disadvantages of reporting past mental problems and treatment.

20. Designate each client to own his own business (related to career goal). Tell him he now must hire staff. Ask him what work habits and traits will he look for in each interview.

21. Ask clients to make up a wish list of activities/hobbies they would like to do when retired. Have them prioritize the list and write steps needed to accomplish their first goal.

22. Have clients write a retirement plan, sharing this with the group. Provide feedback to all members regarding benefits and if plan is realistic and can be accomplished. Reinforce all participation as it occurs.

23. Contact retired business association, have guest speaker talk on subject of retirement--advantages and disadvantages.

# Bibliography

Allen, C. K. (1988). Occupational therapy: Functional assessment of the severity of mental disorders. *Hospital and Community Psychiatry, 39,* 140-142.

Allen, C. K. (1985). *Occupational Therapy for Psychiatric Diseases: Measurement and Management of Cognitive Disabilities.* Boston: Little, Brown.

American Psychiatric Association. (1987). *Diagnostic & Statistical Manual of Mental Disorders* (3rd ed.). Washington, DC: American Psychiatric Association.

American Red Cross. (1988). *American Red Cross Back Injury Prevention: Protect Your Back.* Publisher.

American Red Cross. (1988). *Instructor's Manual.* Town: Publisher.

Anthony, W. A., & Jansen, M. A. (1984). Predicting the vocational capacity of the chronic mentally ill. *American Psychologist, 39,* 537-544.

Asher, I. E. (1989). *An Annotated Index of Occupational Therapy Evaluation Tools.* The American Occupational Therapy Association.

Bethesda Lutheran Home. (1985). *Task Analysis.* Watertown, WI: Bethesda Lutheran Home.

Bruininks, R. H., Woodcock, R. W., Weatherman, R. F., & Hill, B. K. (1984). *Scales of Independent Behavior.* DLM Teaching Resources.

Carroll, I., & Williams, J. (1982). Functional assessment in partial hospitalization: Clinical and administrative applications and implications after one year's utilization of Farmington Functional Assessment Scale. *International Journal of Partial Hospitalization, 1,* 327-339.

Clark, E. N. (1984). *Scoreable Self-care Evaluation* Thorofare, NJ: Slack, Inc.

Canaan, R. A., Blankertz, L., Messinger, K., & Gardner, J. R. (1989). Psychosocial rehabilitation: Towards a theoretical base. *Psychosocial Rehabilitation Journal, 13,* 33-55.

Denton, P. (1988). Assessing the patient's functional performance. *Hospital and Community Psychiatry, 39,* 935-936.

Dunn, W. & McGourty, L. (1989) Application of uniform terminology to practice. *The American Journal of Occupational Therapy, 43*(12),817-831.

Fabian, E. (1989). Work and the quality of life. *Psychosocial Rehabilitation Journal, 12,* 39-49.

Fine, S. B. (1980). Psychiatric treatment and rehabilitation: What's in a name? *National Association of Private Psychiatric Hospitals, 11,* 8-13.

Franklin, J. L., Kittredge, L. D., & Thrasher, D. H. (1975). A survey of factors related to mental hospital admissions. *Hospital and Community Psychiatry, 26,* 749-751.

Hatfield, A. B. Serving the unserved in community rehabilitation programs. *Psychosocial Rehabilitation Journal, 13,* 71-82.

International Association of Psychosocial Rehabilitation Services, Board of Directors. (1985). Psychosocial rehabilitation: Definition, principles and description. *International Association of Psychosocial Rehabilitation Services.* Columbia, Maryland: International Association of Psychosocial Rehabilitation Services.

Jacobs, H. E., Kardashian, S., Kreinbring, R. K., Ponder, R., & Simpson, A. R. (1984). A skills oriented model for facilitating employment among psychiatrically disabled persons. *Rehabilitation Counseling Bulletin, 28,* 87-96.

Landau, S. G., Neal, D. L., Meisner, M., & Prudic, J. (1980). Depressive symptomology among laid off workers. *Journal of Psychiatric Treatment and Evaluation, 2,* 5-12.

Leonardelli, C. A. (1988). *The Milwaukee Evaluation of Daily Living Skills.* Thorofare, NJ: Slack, Inc.

Liberman, R. P. (Ed.) (1988). *Psychiatric Rehabilitation of Chronic Mental Patients.* Washington, DC: American Psychiatric Press, Inc.

Liberman, R. P., Mueser, K. T., Wallace, C. J., Jacobs, H. E., Eckman, T., & Massel, H. K. (1986). Training skills in the psychiatrically disabled: Learning coping and competence. *Schizophrenia Bulletin, 12* (4), 631-647.

McArthur, M. (1989). *Providing Services to Adults with Mental Illness.* Training conference by Michigan Department of Mental Health, Lansing, MI.

Morrison, E., Fisher, L. Y., Wilson, H. S., & Underwood, P. (1985). Nursing adaptation evaluation. *Journal of Psychosocial Nursing, 23,* 10-13.

Palmer, F. (1989). The place of work in psychiatric rehabilitation. *Hospital and Community Psychiatry, 40,* 222-224.

Parnicky, J. J., & Agin, D. (1975). *Pathways Toward Independence.* Columbus: Ohio State University.

Perfetti, L. J., & Bingham, W. C. (1983). Unemployment and self-esteem in metal refinery workers. *Vocational Guidance Quarter 31,* 195 202.

Peterson, C. Q. (1988). Prevocational assessments in mental health. In B. Hemphill (Ed.), *Mental Health Assessment in Occupational Therapy.* Thorofare, NJ: Slack, Inc.

Pratt, H. D. (1989). *Writing Effective Behavioral Goals and Objectives.* Paper presented at Focus 89, Cedar, MI.

Pratt, H. D., Werner, P. C., Austin, P., Loukas, K. L., & Smith, P., (Eds.). (1988). *Goals and Objectives Training Manual* (1st & 2nd eds.). Kalamazoo, MI: Kalamazoo Regional Psychiatric Hospital Printing Services.

Reed, K. L., & Sanderson, S. R. (1983). *Concepts of Occupational Therapy.* Baltimore: Williams & Wilkins.

Rubin, S. & Roessler, R. (1978). Guidelines for successful vocational rehabilitation of the psychiatrically disabled. *Rehabilitation Literature, 38,* 70-74.

Strauss, J. S. (1986). Discussion: What does rehabilitation accomplish? *Schizophrenia Bulletin, 12,* 720-723.

United States Pharmacopoeial Drug Information (1988). *Advice for the Patient.* Volume II. Town: United States Pharmacopoeial Convention, Inc.

Vargas, J. S. (1972). *Writing Worthwhile Behavioral Objectives.* New York: Harper & Row.

Vorspan, R. (1988). Activities of daily living in the clubhouse: You can't vacuum in a vacuum. *Psychosocial Rehabilitation Journal, 12,* 15-21.

Waley, Malott R., & Garcia, M. E., (in press). *Elementary Principles of Behavior.* (2nd ed.). Town: Publisher.

Wallace, C. J., & Liberman, R. P. (1985). Social skills training for patients with schizophrenia. *Psychiatry Research, 15*, 239-237.

*Webster's New World Dictionary* (2nd ed.). (1984). Cleveland: William Collins & World Publishing.

Wong, S. E., Wright, J., Terranova, M. D., Bowen, L., & Zarate, R. (1988). Effects of structured ward activities on appropriate and psychotic behavior of chronic psychiatric patients. *Behavioral Residential Treatment, 3,* 41-50.

Wong, S. E., Terranova, M. D., Bowen, L., Zarate, R., Massel, H. K., & Liberman, R. P. (1987). Providing independent recreational activities to reduce stereotypic vocalizations in chronic schizophrenics. *Journal of Applied Behavior Analysis, 20,* 77-81.

# Index